Gay, Gray, & Fit after 50

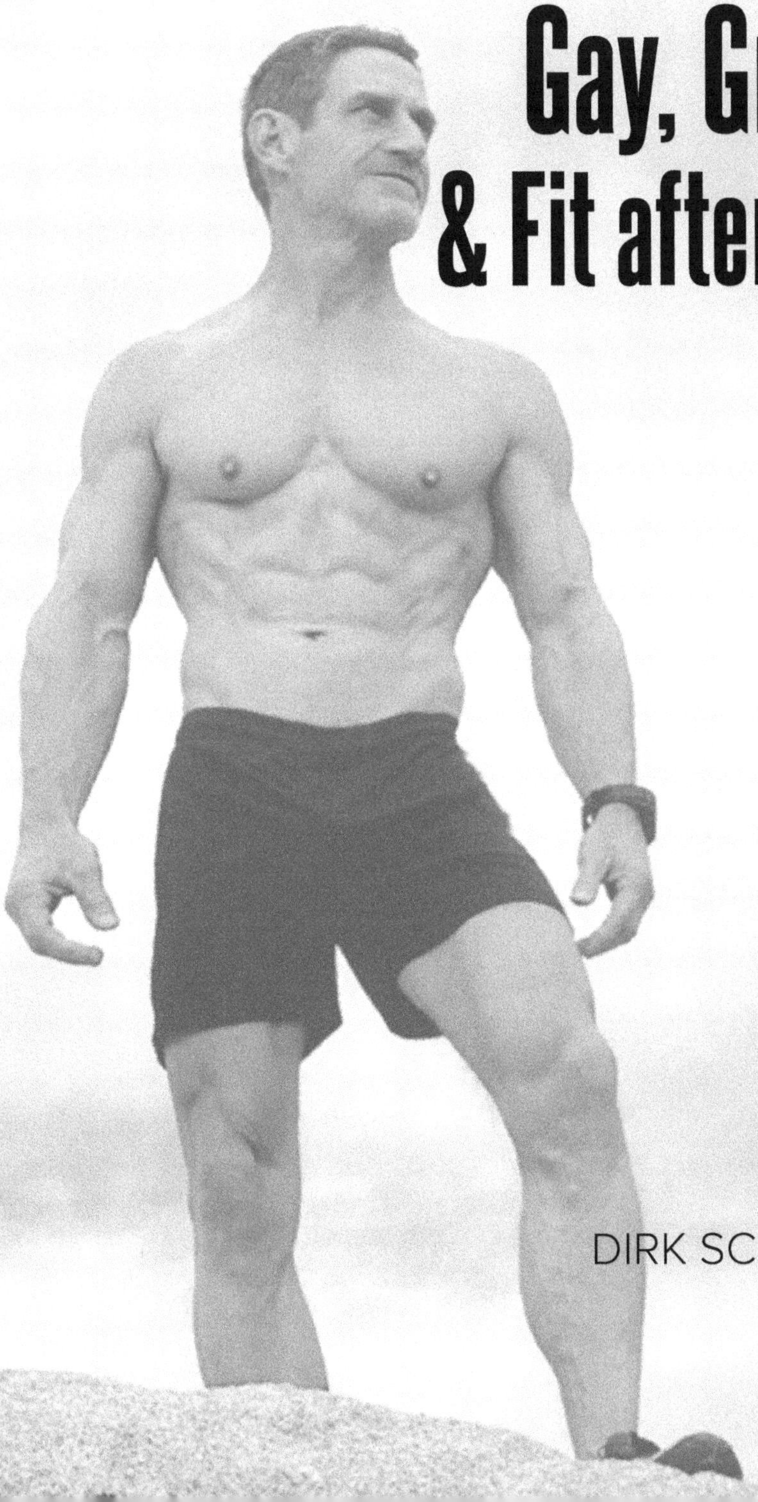

DIRK SCHULTZ

ISBN Paperback: 979-8-9900832-0-2
ISBN eBook: 979-8-9900832-1-9

First Edition
Version 06.2024 | June 2024
Series: M3 Series

Published by: M3 Holistic Media LLC
Palm Springs, California
Email: M3HolisticMedia@gmail.com

Editor: Book Your Brand LLC | David Strauss

DEDICATED TO...

All the Gay Men and women who have come before me who were brave and courageous and helped pave the way for LGBTQ rights, allowing me to be able to write this book comfortably, freely, and safely.

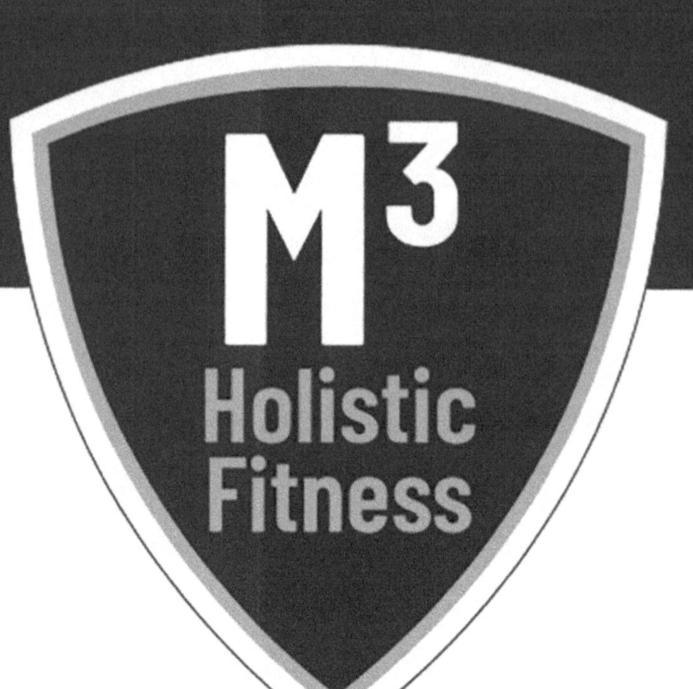
M³
Holistic
Fitness

DISCLAIMER

The material presented in this book is intended for informational and entertainment purposes only. It is not meant to replace professional health or medical advice, diagnosis, or treatment. The author, publisher and any associated parties are not healthcare providers and make no representations or warranties of any kind, either express or implied, concerning the efficacy, appropriateness, or suitability of any healthcare treatments, products, or lifestyle changes.

If you have a pre-existing medical condition, are under medical treatment, or are taking medications, you must consult a qualified healthcare provider for personalized medical advice. Any lifestyle changes, including but not limited to diet and exercise regimens, should only be undertaken under the guidance of a healthcare professional.

By continuing to read this book, you acknowledge and agree that the author, publisher, and any associated parties shall not be liable for any direct, indirect, consequential, special, exemplary, or other damages arising from the application or misapplication of the information contained herein.

Your health is of the utmost importance. Although this book aims to provide helpful insights and tips, it should not be considered a substitute for individualized medical care from a qualified healthcare provider.

By proceeding beyond this point, you indicate your understanding and acceptance of these terms.

CONTENTS

MEET DIRK **11**

GRAND NEW FRONTIER **15**

TECTONIC SHIFT **17**

PART 01. MINDSET · MOVEMENT · MEALS **21**
  DISCOVERING THE M3 METHOD.. 22

PART 02. MINDSET **29**
  M·I·N·D·S·E·T 31
  MINDSET 32
  ANCHOR 1 — VISION 39
  ANCHOR 2 — RELATIONSHIPS 41
  ANCHOR 3 — MINDFUL PRACTICE 44
  ANCHOR 4 — CREATIVITY 50
  ANCHOR 5 — WORK-LIFE BALANCE 53
  ANCHOR 6 — FINANCIAL FITNESS 56
  ANCHOR 7 — STRESS BUSTERS 59
  S.T.R.E.S.S.. 61

PART 03. MOVEMENT **69**
  M·O·V·E·M·E·N·T 70
  GET OFF YOUR ASS! 72
  SUNRISE TO SUNSET.. 112

PART 04. MEALS **127**
  M·E·A·L·S.. 128
  MEALS 130
  THE 5 ELEMENTS OF MEALS 135

ON THE PLATE · OFF THE PLATE. **147**

ON THE PLATE ... 149
    F.O.O.D. ... 150

OFF THE PLATE ... 153
    OVERALL ENVIRONMENT ... 154

YOUR VIBRANT JOURNEY ... 161

BADASS LIFE ... 169
    CREATING YOUR BADASS LIFE ... 169
    B.A.D.A.S.S. ... 171
    A · C · T · I · O · N ... 173

CELEBRATE YOUR NEW REFLECTION ... 175
RECAP OF THE M3 METHOD ... 179
FOUR M3 AGREEMENTS ... 181
FINAL MESSAGE FROM DIRK ... 187
JOURNAL ... 189
    INTRODUCING THE M3 JOURNAL ... 189

ACKNOWLEDGMENTS ... 193
SPECIAL THANKS! ... 197
AN ENDORSEMENT FROM TONY C. ... 199
DIRK'S M3 BLOG ... 203
    BLOG DEFYING THE MYTHS OF AGING ... 204
    BLOG LIFE REIMAGINED ... 207

AUTHOR ... 211
    ABOUT DIRK SCHULTZ ... 211

WELCOME TO...
THE FABULOUS 5TH FLOOR...

YOUR 50s!

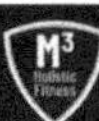

"WHO SAYS YOUR PRIME HAS TO END AT 49?"

Strap in because you're not just crossing into another decade; you're stepping into a golden renaissance of self-discovery, transformation, and—wait for it—sizzling sex appeal! Being a badass gay man over 50 isn't a footnote; it's a headliner.

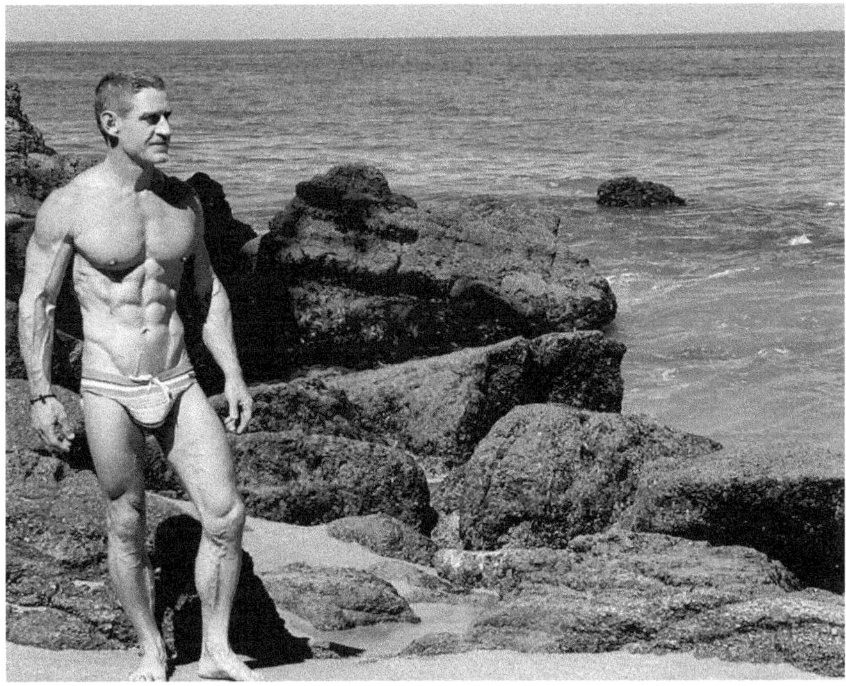

With this book as your ultimate guide, we're diving deep into a journey about way more than just "aging gracefully."

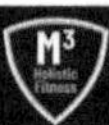

You'll rediscover your inner swagger, reignite your mojo, and boost your confidence until it's off the charts. Trust me, you'll feel as irresistible as a glass of fine wine that's just hit its peak.

Picture this: a life bursting with vitality, oozing charisma, and radiating personal pride. Yeah, that's right—those are the stakes here. Through the lens of M3 Holistic Fitness and the M3 Method, we are carving out a path to emotional resilience, internal peace, and holistic health. This isn't just about 'health' in the traditional sense; we're talking about redefining what it means to be a vibrant, empowered gay man at this stage in your life.

So, are you ready to reclaim your relevance? To turn heads and break hearts (in the best way possible)? To flex your intellectual and emotional muscles as much as your physical ones? You bet you are!

Forget "over the hill." We're scaling the summit, planting our flag, and making this a view to die for. Life starts at 50; you're just getting warmed up. This journey will be filled with enlightenment, empowerment, and a lot of fabulousness.

Let's get this party started!

~Dirk Schultz

Founder | M3 Holistic Fitness | The M3 Method

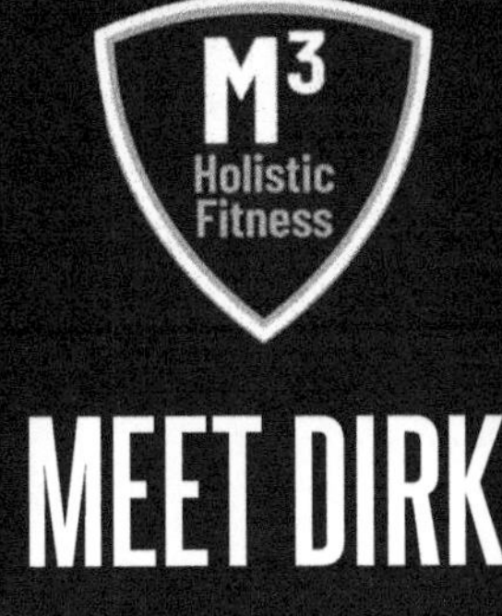

MEET DIRK

"My passion is to help others shift their perspective, rewrite their stories, and build the body and life they've always wanted."
—Dirk Schultz

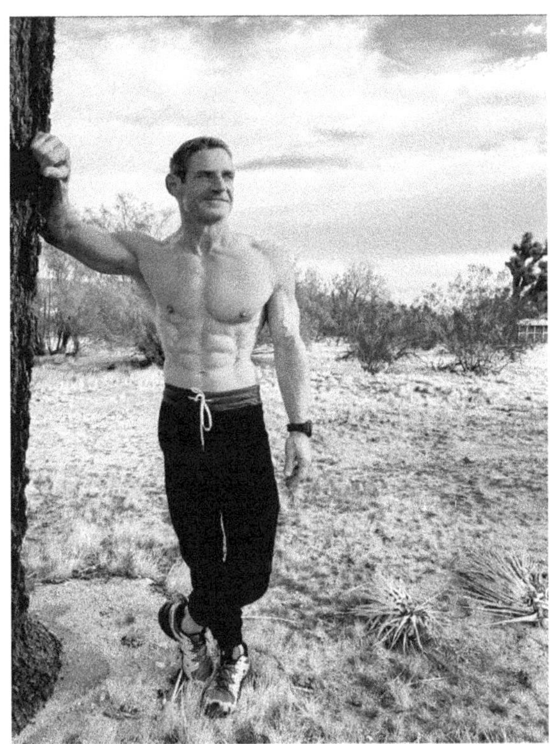

Crossing into my 50s as a gay man, my life experiences profoundly shaped my journey. Having endured a turbulent childhood riddled with abuse and abandonment, fitness served as my sanctuary, a coping mechanism that stood as an external emblem of strength. But as I delved into my past and untangled the complicated narratives I had built, I realized that fitness had evolved for me—it had transitioned from merely an external show of strength to an intimate path of inner work and empowerment. This transformation led me towards a life where I am now free from the hauntings of my past.

For many gay men like me, fitness acts as both a protective shield and an empowering sword. In a community that highly values youth, maintaining an attractive physique often comes more naturally in our younger years. But what happens when you reach the "5th floor" of life, where the end seems nearer than the beginning? How do we reclaim our appeal while embracing the years we've lived?

As I've matured, so have my values, needs, and relationships. The recurring theme in my conversations with other 50+ gay men is consistent: How do we regain our sense of importance and rekindle our social and sexual appeal? It's a real challenge.

Despite being part of a resilient and supportive gay community, the ultimate responsibility for our health rests on our shoulders. Coaches and trainers can only do so much; your true mental and physical transformation requires personal investment. And here's the silver lining—it's an engaging, even enjoyable journey when you have the proper structure and accountability in place.

This brings me to the M3 Method, a holistic fitness philosophy that stands as the cornerstone of M3 Holistic Fitness. Refined throughout my career in the health and fitness industry, the M3 Method initially served as my fitness roadmap.

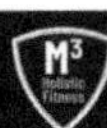

Over time, it has blossomed into a comprehensive lifestyle approach that benefits people from all walks of life. Proper fitness isn't just a physical endeavor; it's a self-reflective journey that starts with a tailored plan addressing the physical, emotional, mental, and spiritual aspects of life. The M3 Method isn't just about building strength; it's about achieving a full-spectrum life transformation. At the core of the M3 Method are three pillars:

Mindset · Movement · Meals.

The path to comprehensive well-being isn't just through your muscles; it's a journey within the trio of these pillars. The M3 Method wellness programs are designed to clear away the obstacles that hinder people from achieving their fullest potential in every aspect of their lives.

With a career in the fitness industry dating back to 2004, including celebrated roles at the Aspen Club and as an Expert Trainer for leading fitness apps, the M3 Method has evolved with my experience and is now as versatile as it is specialized. In addition to my extensive experience, I hold certifications from the Institute for Integrated Nutrition, The Coaches Training Institute, and the National Academy of Sports Medicine, making me uniquely qualified to offer industry-leading specialized training.

Whether you're a fitness newbie or a competitive athlete, my mission is to guide those who are ready to live life on their own terms. After all, if you want to improve your life, you must consistently make changes with strategy, intention, and metrics. The M3 Method will get you there.

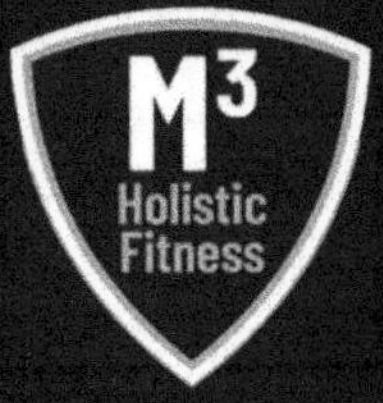

GRAND NEW FRONTIER

Imagine standing at the edge of this grand new frontier of your life; you're now in your 50s and wondering what this next chapter will look like. What do you do? Where do you go? What is and is not working? As these questions circulate in your mind, you realize there is nowhere to go to understand how to navigate this next chapter of your life—until now.

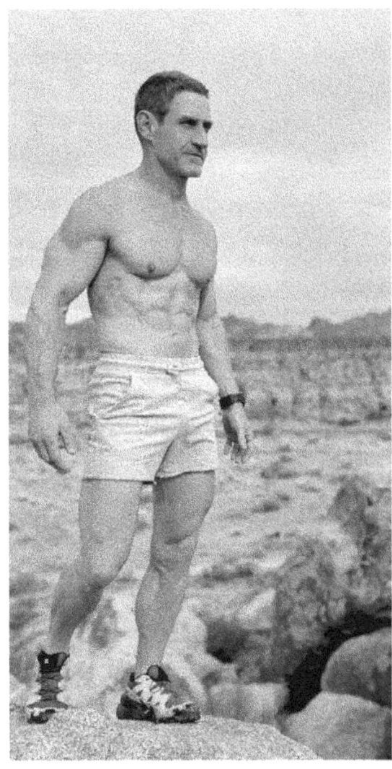

You're not just holding a book—you're gripping the steering wheel of your own personal 50+ revolution. Think of this as less of a 'how-to' guide and more of a 'why not' manifesto for the 50+ gay man. You, my friend, are in the driver's seat, and the open road of untapped possibilities stretches ahead. Forget the stale notion that turning 50 is a step toward social oblivion. This book rips that myth to shreds. Picture instead a vibrant background splashed with electric colors, illustrating how your 50s could be a renaissance of exuberance, sensual pleasure, and charisma so irresistible you'd give your 20-year-old self a run for his money.

Let's talk walls. Society loves to build them around aging—sealing you into 'over the hill' categories or 'past your prime.' But this book? Think of it as your personal wrecking ball. It doesn't just demolish these societal barriers; it dynamites them into confetti. Turning 50 isn't about blending into the grayscale background of mediocrity or learned helplessness; it's your time to burst onto the scene in high-definition technicolor.

If you're expecting some humdrum advice about aging gracefully, think again. This isn't just holistic—it's electric. It's like an inner sparkler that adds years to your life and life to your years, filling each day with vigor and a dash of pizzazz.

So, as you eagerly turn the pages, remember: You're diving headfirst into an ocean of wisdom. You're not merely absorbing text; you're embarking on a transformative voyage that will light up the path to a life so radiantly fulfilling it's like capturing lightning in a bottle. This journey is your golden ticket to unabashedly embracing your 50+ glory, painting each day with hues of excitement and endless energy.

So go ahead and enjoy this rollercoaster of a ride—you're in for the journey of a lifetime.

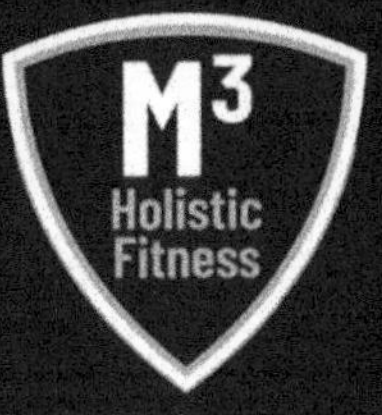

TECTONIC SHIFT

When the clock strikes midnight on the eve of their 50th birthday, many gay men feel a tectonic shift—a rumbling eruption of emotions of uncertainty and surprise. It's not just a milestone; it's an awakening. Suddenly, a golden age is staring back at us that only moments ago seemed years away, and it comes bearing gifts of unique experiences and untold challenges. Yet, as we step over this threshold, we must embrace these realities with humility and vigor to lead vibrant, fulfilling lives as gay men in our 50s and beyond.

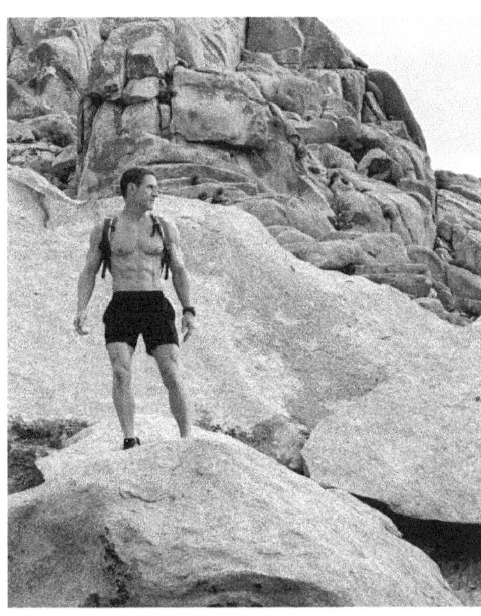

At this juncture, health stops being a whisper and starts to shout. It becomes an insistent companion, prompting us to look into the eyes of medical concerns that cast their shadows over our once-youthful lives. The ugly face of aching joints, slowing metabolism, and hormonal imbalances that make us retire our favorite jeans and destabilize our energy and mood become all too familiar. As these realities settle in, routine health check-ups move from the back seat to the cockpit. But the medical demands extend beyond the physical. Our mental and emotional well-being also takes a new direction as we place a higher value on closer relationships and less weight on casual connections.

Exercise also demands more of our attention. Gone are the days when maintaining fitness was a breeze. Now, it's a commitment requiring a tailored strategy that adapts our routines to match our evolving physical capacities, understanding that the right activities can rejuvenate our bodies and spirits. Whether it's the calming energy of yoga, the dynamic pulse of swimming, or the raw power of weightlifting, the activity that resonates with us becomes more than a routine; it becomes a lifeline.

When we hit 50, society's infatuation with youth can make us feel sidelined, as though we've been dealt a bad hand in a high-stakes game. But what's easily overlooked is the royal flush we already hold—years filled with irreplaceable experiences and wisdom that youth can't buy. Strong social networks within the LGBTQ+ community turn from mere social embellishments to essential lifelines, empowering us against isolation and giving us platforms to connect, validate, and celebrate each other's lives.

Amidst these shifts, self-care evolves from an optional indulgence to a non-negotiable priority. This isn't just about pampering spa days; it's about supporting our physical, emotional, and mental selves in a manner that fuels us to face whatever comes our way. Stigmas and biases related to our

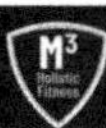

age and sexual orientation might try to derail us, but we rise above them armed with self-compassion, boundaries, and joyful activities.

Turning 50+ isn't an end; it's a renaissance—a blend of the wisdom accumulated from the past and the potential for future discovery. By seizing control of our health, fine-tuning our approach to fitness, and developing rich social bonds, we create a new frontier to flourish during this next stage of our lives.

This does not have to be a solo expedition as we wade through these changes. The M3 Method is your companion, a compass guiding you through the unique obstacles and opportunities that come with being a gay man over 50. It's more than just words on a page; it's a declaration that we can survive this new chapter of our lives and thrive in it. It begins with understanding the relationship between Mindset, Movement, and Meals.

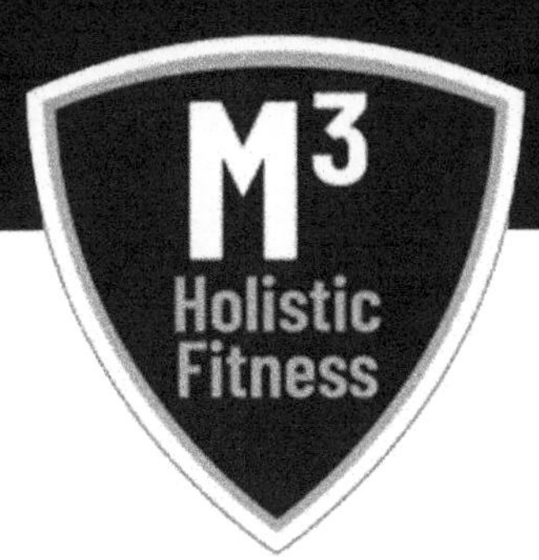

PART ONE

MINDSET · MOVEMENT · MEALS

Discovering The M3 Method

The M3 Method is about quality of life—not just about physical vitality, but the freedom to enjoy simple pleasures, like leisurely dinners with your closest friends, adventurous travel, an enriching social life, and a hot date with "you know who."

When you cross the BIG-5-0 threshold, it's like your body starts sending you invoices for past neglect. Those aches in your joints are not random; they're wake-up calls. Your metabolism decides it's on a casual stroll, not a sprint, making weight gain an unsolicited guest. And let's not forget the energy drop; it's like someone turned the wattage down on your inner light bulb.

And then there's the waning libido and ambition—it's like they packed up and went on a hiatus. These are not just quirks of aging; they're your body's flashing red lights signaling that a holistic overhaul is needed ASAP. That's where the M3 Method steps in. It's not a wellness fad or trend—it's an absolute must for preserving and enhancing the quality of every facet of your life.

As a gay man in my 50s, I understand the unique challenges that come with this stage of life. That's why I'm all about Holistic Fitness—a lifestyle that looks at you as an entire package, not just a set of body parts. Think of it like this: A gardener doesn't just water one flower in a garden; they nurture every plant. Holistic Fitness works the same way. It's about understanding that your health, happiness, and how long you live are all tied together.

Every part of you needs some TLC to feel and be truly well. And that's where the M3 Method comes in. It's the backbone of Holistic Fitness, focusing on the three main pillars of Mindset, Movement, and Meals. Nail these three, and you're setting yourself up to live a bold, beautiful, BADASS life.

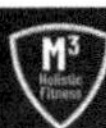

MINDSET

Mindset is the beliefs and attitudes shaping how we perceive and respond to life's challenges and opportunities. It's not just an internal monologue; it's the lens through which we view the world and our approach to everything, including movement and meals. With our mindset, we have either positive or negative expectations for life. With a growth-oriented mindset, we can transform obstacles into avenues for personal development, instilling a sense of positivity that fuels our determination. Focusing on progress over perfection, challenges become learning opportunities.

MOVEMENT

Movement isn't merely exercise—it's the vibrant pulse that courses through our everyday lives. Far beyond the four walls of a gym, movement encompasses anything from high-octane workouts to soul-soothing yoga sessions, from expressive dancing to leisurely walks that let your mind wander. It's the antidote to modern life's sedentary nature, an electric charge that powers up your body and mind. But it does even more: it pumps endorphins through your system, boosting your mood and melting stress away.

Regular movement improves not just your physique but also your mental acuity, sharpening focus and enhancing memory. It plays a crucial role in emotional well-being, too, helping to dispel anxiety and ignite a sense of inner peace. Simply put, movement is a comprehensive package for better living—it enlivens your spirit, strengthens your body, and sharpens your mind, making every day more dynamic and fulfilling.

MEALS

Meals are far more than just the food on your plate; they represent a holistic approach to nourishment that caters to our physical, emotional, and spiritual needs. The 'On the Plate' aspect focuses on balanced, nutritious eating that fuels our bodies. In contrast, the 'Off the Plate' dimension includes other forms of nourishment like relationships and our surrounding environment. Meals are not just about sustenance for our bodies but also for our souls, combining both the tangible and intangible aspects that feed our spirit.

The M3 Method is more than a wellness program; it's a holistic blueprint for achieving both physical fitness and emotional, mental, and spiritual health. This approach encourages you to live consciously, immersing yourself fully in each moment while being mindful of what you put in your mind and body.

For gay men who have hit the 50-year milestone, the M3 Method is more than just helpful—it's truly transformative. It helps you organize your daily routine and make conscious lifestyle decisions. You can take on the challenge independently or involve others in your community.

In a society that prizes youth and physical attractiveness, the M3 Method is a much-needed path to peace of mind, especially as you face the unique challenges of aging without kids and perhaps with a dwindling social circle. As loneliness concerns loom, the M3 Method is your go-to roadmap, enhancing your quality of life as you journey through your 50s and beyond.

The dynamic interplay among the M3 Method's three core pillars—Mindset, Movement, and Meals—is vividly illustrated in the following diagram:

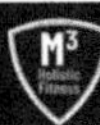

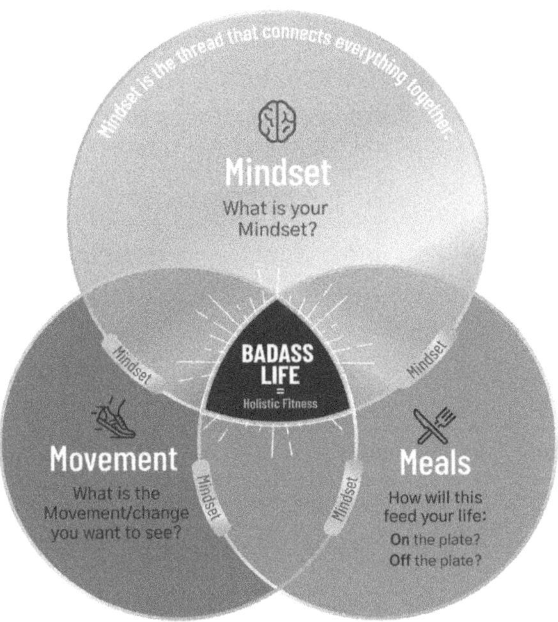

Each element is a standalone powerhouse, but their synergy propels your wellness to the next level. This cooperative interaction sets the stage for a holistic transformation that transcends a basic health plan; it's a full-scale lifestyle overhaul that seamlessly integrates physical, mental, and spiritual aspects of your entire life.

Starting your journey with the M3 Method is a long-term commitment built upon a focus that thrives on continual growth. As you traverse the path to holistic health, you'll learn to cherish each moment and celebrate every achievement, big or small.

Remember, the road to ultimate wellness isn't just a straight shot or a dull stroll; it's a rollercoaster ride full of scenic routes, peaks, valleys, and eye-popping vistas. The M3 Method is your co-pilot on this thrilling journey, serving as your all-in-one toolkit for life enhancement. It arms you with a rock-solid Mindset to conquer challenges, revs you up with Movement that energizes every fiber of your being, and satisfies your soul with Meals that go beyond mere calories. Within this dynamic framework, each step you take isn't just incremental progress; it's a turbo boost that elevates your entire quality of life. So, buckle up, and let's make this ride an exhilarating one!

As your eyes glide over the M3 Circle of Life diagram below, you'll notice it's sliced into three delicious pie sections: Mindset, Movement, and Meals. Each slice is jam-packed with specifics to dive into. That's precisely how this book is structured and designed to roll. So, let's cut ourselves a piece of that pie and start feasting on life-enhancing wisdom!

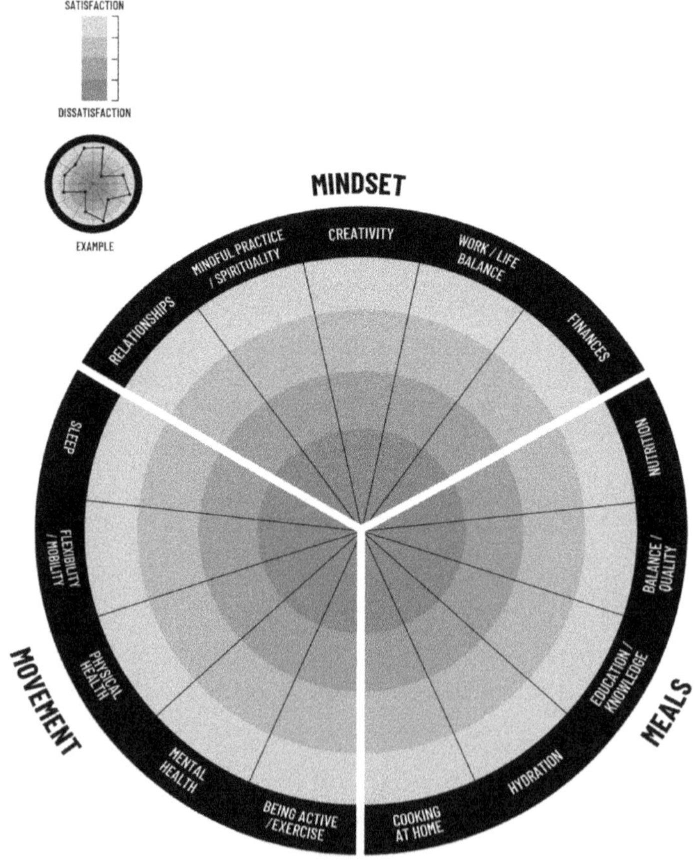

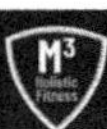

Imagine This: A life where your Mindset, Movement, and Meals seamlessly blend, each one amplifying the others. It's more than just a healthy lifestyle; it's a state of effortless flow enriched with purpose and intention. In this reality, your mental clarity influences your physical activity, nourishing your dietary choices. It's a harmonious cycle where every element is dialed in, and the result is a version of you optimized for joy, wellness, and meaningful connections.

As you journey through this book, we will delve into the unique sub-elements that form each of the three M3 pillars. This will equip you with a comprehensive toolbox for crafting a life that's both good and extraordinary.

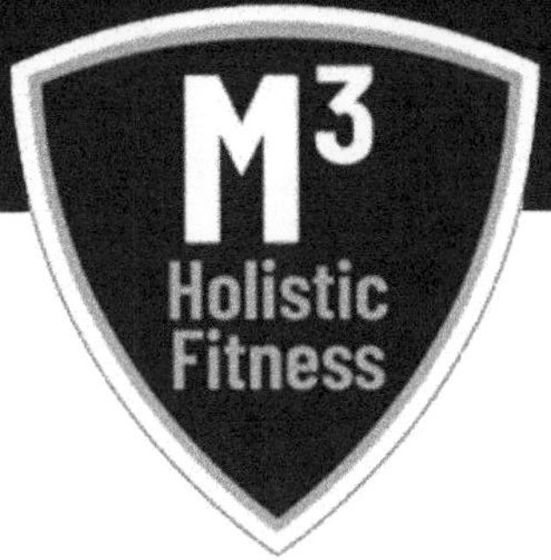

PART TWO

MINDSET

*"The only thing that stands between you
and the life you've always wanted... is you."*
—Dirk Schultz

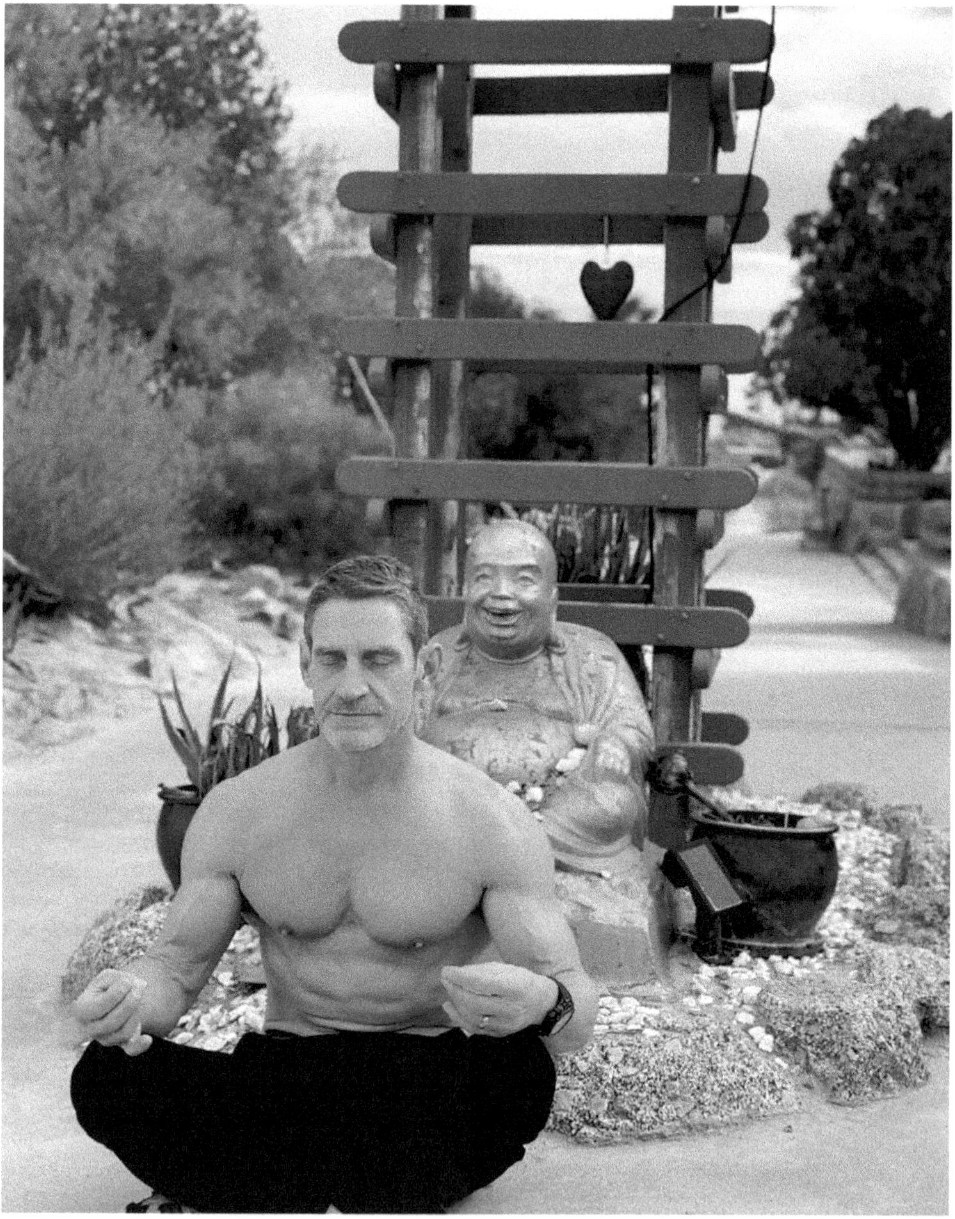

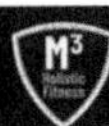

M·I·N·D·S·E·T

M | Mindfulness: The practice of fully engaging in the present moment. This involves setting aside distractions and focusing on what you are experiencing, helping reduce stress and enhance peace of heart and mind.

I | Intention: Setting clear, positive, and attainable goals. It involves focusing on what you want to achieve and ensuring all your actions align with those goals.

N | Nourishment: Providing your body with the nutrients it needs to function at its best. It also extends to nourishing your mind with positive thoughts and experiences.

D | Determination: This is about persisting despite obstacles and setbacks. It's about committing to your goals and doing whatever it takes to achieve them.

S | Self Awareness: Recognizing and understanding your emotions, strengths, weaknesses, and behaviors. It's about understanding how others perceive you and how your actions and attitudes affect them.

E | Empathy: This means understanding and sharing the feelings of others. Empathy allows you to build strong, positive relationships and better understand the people around you.

T | Tenacity: The determination to continue trying even when things get tough. It's about not giving up when you face challenges and having the resilience to keep going.

Mindset

The Cornerstone of the M3 Method

"Genetics loads the gun, and lifestyle pulls the trigger."
~Mehmet Oz

Why is mindset the starting point for your holistic health journey? Because your mindset, how you think and interact with each day, is the foundational thread that ties every aspect of your life together. It isn't just the backbone; it's the entire framework supporting your capacity for resilience, stability, and navigating life's intricate maze. It's about establishing an internal environment that empowers you—a lens through which you perceive and engage with the world. It's crafting an inner dialogue that reinforces your ability to make wise choices and view challenges as opportunities for growth rather than insurmountable setbacks.

Imagine your mindset as a personalized roadmap, guiding your interactions with the world around you. It's the gentle push that encourages you to lace up your sneakers even on low-energy days, the spark of inspiration that leads you to choose a nutrient-packed salad over a bag of chips, and the driving force that helps you strike a harmonious work-life balance.

Your mindset becomes the invisible engine propelling you toward your goals, urging you to become the best version of yourself. Cultivating such a focused and uplifting mindset isn't just advantageous—it's essential for achieving holistic health and a life filled with profound satisfaction.

Now, let's explore the crucial difference between a positive and negative mindset. Your mindset, whether positive or negative, significantly impacts your overall well-being.

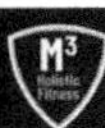

A positive mindset is like having a good friend who always sees the silver lining—it keeps you going when times get tough, encourages you to take healthy risks, and helps you find opportunities even in bad situations. It's the internal pep talk that says, 'You've got this,' when you're facing challenges.

On the flip side, a negative mindset is like that naysayer friend who's always bringing you down. It fills your head with doubts, holds you back from trying new things, and makes everything feel more challenging than it has to be. It's the voice saying, 'This will never work when facing an obstacle.

But what's even more remarkable is how your overall mindset ripples through various dimensions of your life, affecting the quality of your health, relationships, social life, and intimacy in profound ways. Allow me to illustrate this with some examples:

Health

A positive mindset often leads to healthier lifestyle choices. When you possess a positive outlook on life, you're more inclined to engage in regular exercise, opt for nutritious foods, and ensure you get adequate rest. This, in turn, can result in improved physical health, increased energy levels, and a strengthened immune system. Conversely, a negative mindset can contribute to stress, which has been linked to various health issues such as high blood pressure, heart disease, and compromised immune function.

Relationships

Your mindset plays a pivotal role in your interactions with others. A positive mindset makes you more open, empathetic, and compassionate in your relationships. It fosters effective communication and equips you to resolve conflicts constructively. In contrast, a negative mindset may lead to misunderstandings, resentment, and strained relationships. People with a negative mindset may find it challenging to trust others, potentially resulting in isolation and a lack of intimacy in their connections.

Social Life

How you perceive the world directly influences your social life. A positive mindset often makes you more outgoing and inclined to engage in social activities. This positivity attracts like-minded individuals who share your optimism, resulting in a vibrant and supportive social network. Conversely, a negative mindset may lead to withdrawal from social interactions, triggering feelings of loneliness and isolation.

Intimacy

Your mindset also impacts intimacy. A positive mindset boosts your confidence, making you feel more desirable and emotionally connected with your partner. This can profoundly enhance the quality of your intimate relationships. A negative mindset may lead to self-doubt, anxiety, and a lack of intimacy, hindering your ability to fully engage in intimate moments with your partner or lovers.

In essence, your mindset is the compass guiding your holistic health journey. And when it comes to fine-tuning that compass for the journey ahead, the M3 Mindset takes focus and intention to a much deeper level.

The M3 Mindset

The M3 Mindset isn't just a passing fad or a buzzword; it's a transformative mental shift that sets in when you come face-to-face with the reality that life's finish line is ever

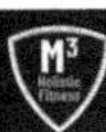

approaching. This realization triggers an unshakable conviction that taking charge of your health and wellness is no longer just a good idea—it's an urgent, non-negotiable must-do. Seamlessly blending an intellectual understanding with a do-or-die urgency, the M3 Mindset transforms your mindset from a "should-do" to a "must-do," making it mission-critical for a life rich in quality and longevity.

The M3 Mindset is far more than a mantra or a health tip; it's a significant reorientation that runs counter to societal norms fixated on quick fixes and immediate gratification. It serves as your battle cry and catalyst, urging you to defy conventional wisdom by making proactive, long-term wellness not just an aspiration but an absolute obligation.

In adopting the M3 Mindset, you're not just dipping your toes into the waters of better living; you're diving headfirst into a set of higher personal standards that can extend your lifespan and enhance the quality of your years. This specialized perspective keeps you asking, 'How do today's choices fit into the M3 Circle of Life?'

At its core, the M3 Mindset houses a growth mindset—a belief that you can continually improve and evolve. This isn't just fluffy, feel-good rhetoric; it's a life-extending practice. Studies have shown that a growth mindset contributes to a healthier mind, higher-quality relationships, and greater longevity.

Adopting the M3 Mindset is a decision to hold yourself to a higher standard of wellness. This choice may go against conventional wisdom or societal norms, particularly in a culture that often prioritizes immediate gratification over long-term health. But the beauty of this mindset lies in its long-term benefits, especially when it comes to longevity.

By adhering to the principles of the M3 Method, you're investing in a lifestyle that may challenge some societal norms but pays dividends in enhancing not just the length but also the quality of your life. This is not just a different way to live; it's a better way to live, providing a robust framework for holistic wellness that stands the test of time. As Wayne Dyer insightfully said, 'When we change how we look at things, the things we look at change.'

To support you in adopting and maintaining your M3 Mindset, I highly recommend incorporating the M3 Mindset Journal into your daily routine. This isn't a typical journal; it's a disciplined practice designed to keep you engaged, accountable, and aligned with your wellness goals. By making it a part of your daily discipline, you can easily track your progress, reflect on your choices, and strategize for the future. Consider the journal your companion and confidant on this holistic journey—a tangible way to stay committed to your higher standard of personal health.

So, let's start this life-extending adventure by adopting an M3 Mindset for the long-term benefits. This way of thinking serves as fertile ground for nurturing a lifestyle that feels good and adds years to your life. Together, we'll draw up your personalized roadmap to M3 Holistic Fitness, a journey defined by a mindset that's not just positive but perpetually evolving.

Implementing the M3 Mindset into your daily life involves a multi-dimensional approach that touches on decision-making, self-questioning, and setting new standards.

Here are some questions to ask yourself that will bring you in alignment with the M3 Mindset.

Daily Questions to Ask Yourself

What are my wellness priorities today?

How do my choices today align with the M3 Circle of Life?

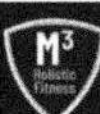

Am I seeking instant gratification or making decisions for long-term wellness?

What can I improve or learn today to grow personally and health-wise?

How am I holding myself accountable for my wellness journey?

Daily Choices

Physical Activity: Choose to be active, even if it's just a 20-minute walk or a quick home workout.

Nutrition: Opt for balanced, nutritious meals that fuel your body and mind rather than quick, unhealthy fixes.

Mental Wellness: Dedicate time to activities that soothe and sharpen your mind such as meditation, reading, or quiet reflection.

Rest: Prioritize quality sleep and downtime to recover and rejuvenate.

Community: Engage with like-minded individuals or groups that support your wellness journey.

Journaling: Record your experiences, feelings, and progress in the M3 Mindset Journal for reflection and accountability.

New Standards to Live By

Non-Negotiable Wellness: Health and well-being are not optional but an urgent priority.

Long-Term over Short-Term: Always opt for choices that contribute to your long-term wellness over immediate but fleeting gratification.

Constant Growth: Never settle for stagnancy. Always look for opportunities to grow mentally, physically, and emotionally.

Accountability: Use tools and resources like the M3 Mindset Journal to hold yourself accountable for your daily actions and long-term goals.

Implementing these elements daily solidifies the M3 Mindset as a cornerstone in your life, steering you toward a more meaningful and sustainable wellness journey.

The Empowering Potential of the M3 Mindset

Embarking on a wellness journey at any age involves more than just counting calories, clocking miles, and eating the right foods. Especially for gay men over 50, it's about nurturing a holistic lifestyle that appreciates life's highs and lows. The M3 Method brings this focus sharply into view with seven anchors designed to harmonize with your overall sense of wholeness.

Vision · Relationships · Mindful Practice · Creativity

Work-Life Balance · Financial Fitness · Stress Busters

These are not just fancy buzzwords; these seven anchors work in synergy. For instance, Work-Life Balance can boost your energy to engage in meaningful Relationships or pursue your Vision. Likewise, Financial Fitness might allow you to delve into creativity or a mindful practice. It's a holistic circle, much like the integrative focus of the M3 Method itself. Now, let's take a closer look at each of the seven anchors.

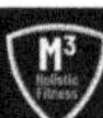

ANCHOR 1 — VISION

V | Visualize what you want: Create a vivid mental picture of what you want, where you want to be, and who you want to be with. Write it down and read it daily with enthusiasm.

I | Intentional action: Take intentional action toward your vision. A vision is a dream without action. Regular, intentional action toward your vision will keep you motivated and moving forward.

S | Say yes or no: Assess if this decision or opportunity in front of you is bringing you closer or further away from the vision you have for your life. If it brings you closer, go for it; if it takes you further away, rethink it.

I | Integrate your values: When a vision aligns with your values, there is a stronger connection to it and more flow in its pursuit.

O | Own your worth: Recognize your value and believe that you deserve the life you want. Challenge self-doubts and fears and prove them wrong.

N | Now is the time: If not now, when? Time will pass whether we like it or not, so decide where you want to be on the other side of it. Now is the time to take action.

Holistic health begins with a clear vision of what you want your health and life to look like. If you want to improve your health meaningfully:

1. Start by figuring out precisely what you're aiming for.

2. Forget the vague goals and the one-size-fits-all diets and workout plans.

3. Think about what a healthy life looks like for you, from your mental state to your physical condition.

Having this clear goal helps you make smarter daily choices, whether in your career, relationships, or even your daily routine.

Before you start counting calories or meditating, take a moment to think about what "being healthy" means for you. Once you've got that sorted, you've got a practical measure for all your big and small decisions. This isn't just about what you eat or how you exercise, but how you live your life day to day.

Writing down these goals can make a big difference, too. Studies show you're 42% more likely to achieve your dreams just by jotting them down. So, grab a pen and get specific. Don't worry about judgment; this is for you. Your written goals become your yardstick, helping you decide if each decision you face is getting you closer or taking you further away from where you want to be.

So, let's get real: if you want to make a lasting change in your health, start by setting a clear and personal vision for what that means. It's more than just a mental exercise; it's an action plan that helps ensure every step you're taking is in the right direction.

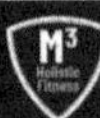

ANCHOR 2 — RELATIONSHIPS

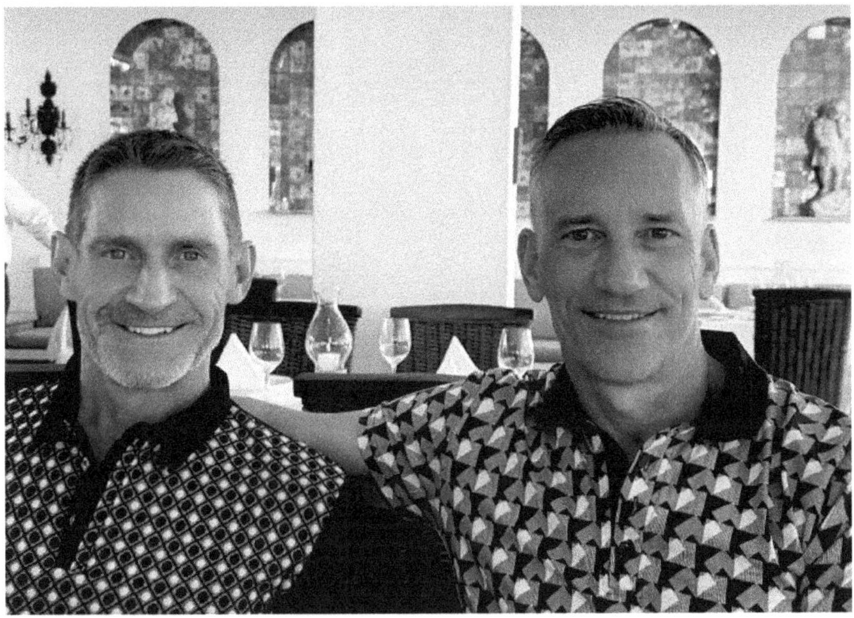

Relationships are absolute game-changers. When they're on point, they lift us to new heights. But let's be real: when they're off, they can pull us into a downward spiral, leaving us stressed, wounded, and lost. According to the M3 Method, no matter the type—social, family, intimate, or professional—relationships should be high-value connections that propel you forward. Especially as we age, it's crucial to audit our close relationships to ensure they align with our goals and values. Time is too precious to waste on connections that hold us back.

Here are ten questions to help you audit your relationships:

1. Does this relationship align with my values and goals?

2. Is there mutual respect and understanding between us?

3. Do we communicate openly and honestly with ourselves and each other?

4. Is this a relationship where I can be my authentic self?

5. Does this connection add positivity and joy to my life?

6. Do I feel supported and uplifted in this relationship?

7. Are boundaries clearly established and respected?

8. Is there a balance of give and take, or is it one-sided?

9. Do we resolve conflicts in a healthy, constructive manner?

10. Do I look forward to spending time with this person?

Developing and maintaining relationships is like gardening. Quality relationships don't just pop up; they require time, attention, and much understanding. You've got to set boundaries, like fencing in your plants. This provides a foundation of mutual respect. Then, you water and nurture the relationship with open communication. But don't forget empathy—just like a gardener understands what a plant needs, you've got to understand the feelings and perspectives of others.

Now, what's the payoff? Strong, healthy relationships light up our lives. They make us happier, more content, and mentally and emotionally better off. Who doesn't want that? This is particularly true for gay men over 50, where good friends are not just lovely to have; they're essential. These people get your jokes, have been there through thick and thin, and make everyday life a bit brighter.

Let's zoom out and talk about your ideal M3 relationships—your community. It's not just about sharing a ZIP code or a hobby; it's about finding your tribe—people who understand you to your core. Within this circle, you're never flying solo, and the value of that is immeasurable. And let's not forget about support. Life has its ups and downs, and when the going gets tough, having a supportive crew makes a world of difference. Whether you're dealing with health issues, fi-

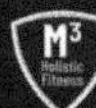

nancial stress, or just the daily grind, friends make the ride smoother.

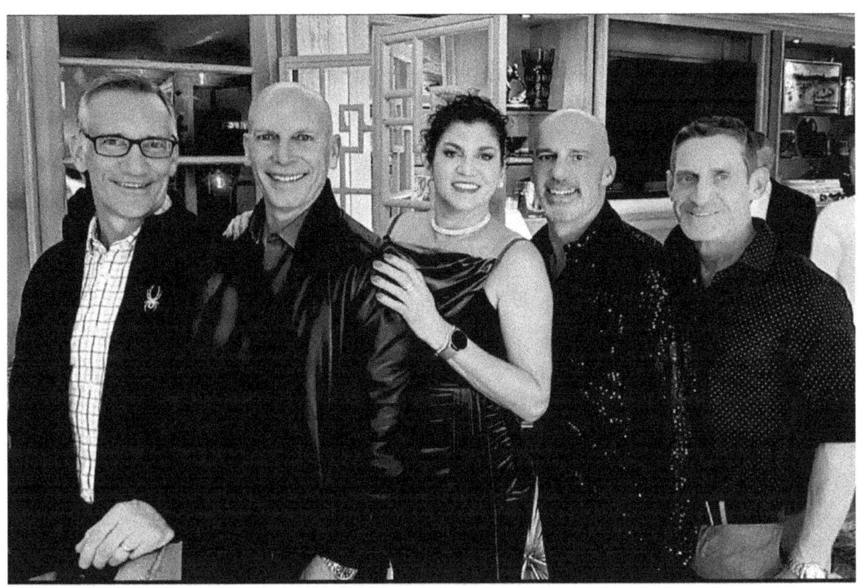

Laughter? Oh, it's the best medicine. Have you ever laughed so hard that it hurt? That's what good friends bring into your life. They turn ordinary days into "remember when" stories.

And traveling with pals? That's the cherry on top. Whether it's road trips or overseas adventures, these shared experiences create memories that last a lifetime.

At the core of all this is trust. It's about being your true self sharing your deepest fears and highest hopes without judgment. This is what makes friendships rich and layered.

So, for gay men over 50, these relationships are not just a nice-to-have; they're a must-have. They offer a sense of belonging, emotional security, loads of laughter, and a vivid canvas to paint life's adventures. They create a space where you can be unapologetically, beautifully you. And really, isn't that what life's all about?

ANCHOR 3 — MINDFUL PRACTICE

Mindfulness and spirituality are not just New Age buzzwords but essential gears in the M3 Method. Think of them as your life's navigational compass and anchor. They guide you towards a balanced mindset and keep you rooted, no matter how turbulent life gets.

So, what's the lowdown? Mindfulness is the practice of being fully engaged in the present moment, not held captive by past regrets or future anxieties. It's like an instant check-in for your mental and emotional state. Remember, it becomes even more important to be mindful of the here and now as we age. We have less time to course-correct, making each moment—and our relationships—infinitely more valuable.

Getting into the nitty-gritty, mindfulness means being intentional with your daily choices, both big and small. Each decision you make, even the seemingly trivial ones, sets the stage for the kind of life you lead. So, being mindful is about tuning into those decisions and understanding their long-term impact.

So, how do you incorporate mindfulness into your daily grind? Start your morning off with a moment of stillness. Take a few minutes to meditate, write in a journal, or recite an affirmation that resonates with you. This brief morning ritual acts like an emotional buffer, giving you a well of tranquility you can dip into throughout the day.

Spirituality is your deeper connection to the essence of who you are and what you believe. It doesn't have to be religious; it could be a connection to nature, art, or community. Spirituality becomes increasingly important for aging gay men, offering a profound sense of belonging and peace amidst life's highs and lows.

So, if you're a gay man over 50 looking to enrich your life through the M3 Method, think of mindfulness and spiritual-

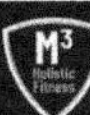

ity as your dynamic duo. They'll offer you emotional stability, mental clarity, and a touch of soulful wisdom. Most importantly, they give you space to be the most authentic version of yourself.

Mindfulness with Self

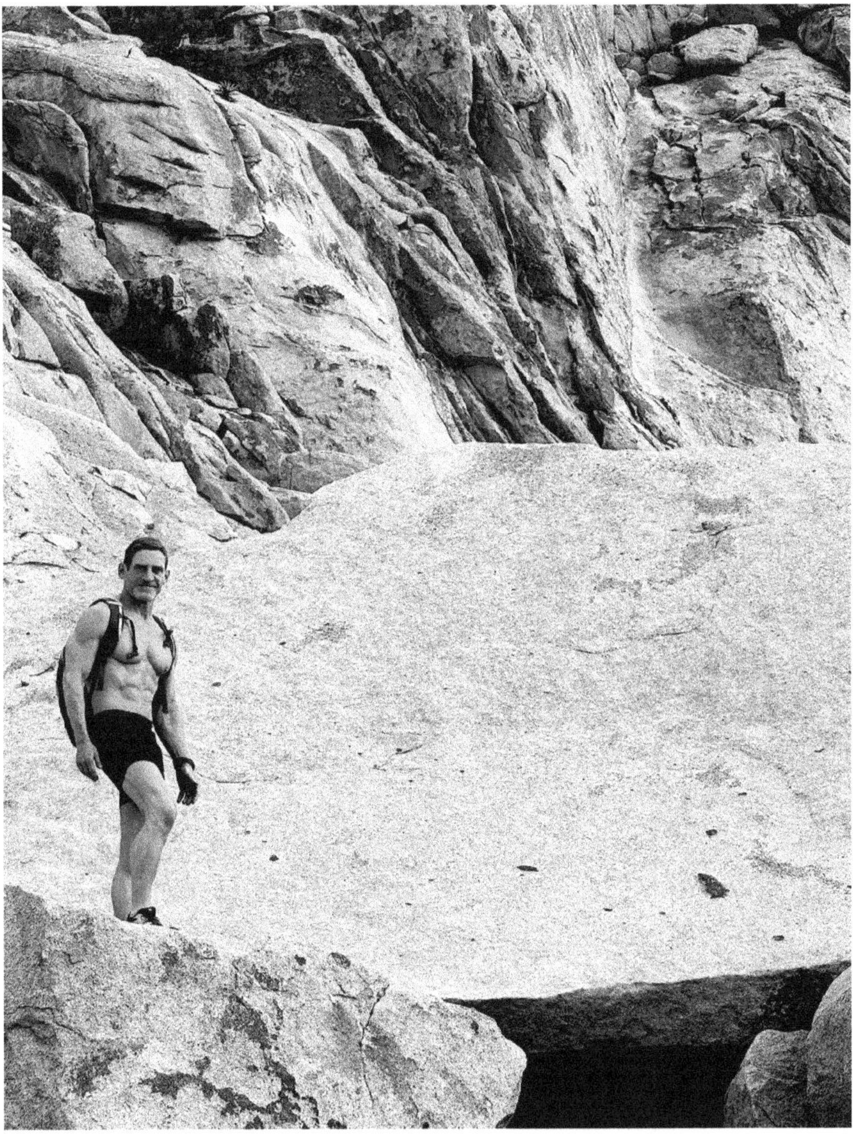

Picture this: You've had one of those grueling days that could make anyone consider early retirement. Meeting after meeting, decision after decision—it's been a marathon. You finally get home, and you're frazzled. Now, the old you might have vegged out in front of the TV or mindlessly scrolled through social media. But you're on the M3 Method now, and you've got a better game plan. Instead, you opt for a mindful timeout.

You settle into your favorite comfy chair or cozy corner and close your eyes. Your focus turns to your breathing: deep, intentional inhales and exhales. As you breathe in, you visualize serenity filling you up. And as you breathe out, you picture all that pent-up stress evaporating into thin air. It's like you're rebooting your emotional system.

You don't run away from your thoughts or feelings; you observe them like clouds passing in the sky. There are no judgments, no "should haves" or "could haves," just acceptance. This pause lets you transition from the whirlwind of your day to a more balanced, relaxed state of mind.

Being a gay man over 50, taking time for yourself isn't just a luxury; it's a must. Aging comes with its challenges, and looking after our emotional well-being is key to staying healthy and nurturing our connections. This peaceful retreat of mindfulness offers the recharge you deserve, allowing you to embrace life with the mantra: "Stay Calm, Stay Cool, Stay Connected."

So, there you have it—a slice of mindfulness, custom-fit to help you handle whatever life throws your way. It's not just about surviving; it's about thriving. And that, my friend, makes all the difference.

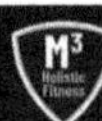

Mindfulness Toward Others

Imagine—you're sitting down with a longtime friend, someone with whom you've probably shared laughs, tears, and plenty of good stories. They start opening up about something that's been weighing them down. Now, given the craziness of life and especially as we age, it's easy to half-listen while your mind wanders elsewhere. Maybe you're tempted to jump in with advice, or your mind drifts to something similar that happened to you.

But wait, you remember the M3 Method. You switch gears and become mindfully present. Your focus narrows down like a laser on what they are saying, how they are saying it, and what they're not saying but feeling. You put all your stuff—thoughts, judgments, the day's distractions—on the shelf for a bit. Your presence says, "I'm here for you and nowhere else."

For us 50+ gay men, this is more than good manners; it's essential. Our friendships are our lifelines and deserve the full richness of our attention. When you give your friend the room to express himself without fear of being judged or interrupted, you're rolling out a red carpet for open, honest communication.

By practicing mindfulness this way, you're not just being a good friend but embodying the M3 Method's principle of high-value connections. You're making the interaction not just a moment in time but a meaningful step toward a deeper journey. That's what it means to be "Calm, Cool, and Connected." And it's not just good for him; it enriches your emotional life, creating a deeper, more empathetic relationship that stands the test of time.

Mindfulness and Spirituality

As you can see, practicing mindfulness can help reduce anxiety, sharpen your emotional intelligence, and make you feel more content with your life. Spirituality is about connecting with something bigger than yourself. It's not necessarily about being religious—though for some people, it certainly could be—but more about a deep-rooted sense of purpose and meaning in your life. Spirituality can take many forms. For some, it might be sitting in quiet meditation or practicing yoga. For others, it might simply mean spending time outdoors, taking in the beauty of nature.

While diverse in its expression, spirituality is rooted in the quest for a deeper understanding of your place in the universe. It's about acknowledging a connection to something larger than yourself, be it a divine entity, the natural world, or the collective human experience. This pursuit of meaning and purpose can be fulfilled through meditation, yoga, time spent in nature, or participation in religious or spiritual communities.

Watch out for habits that may detract from your mindfulness and spirituality. Excessive screen time, involvement in negative or gossipy conversations, and a lack of self-care can all disrupt your mindful practices. Creating boundaries around these behaviors, as you would with a harmful relationship, can help preserve your mental and emotional well-being.

These mindful and spiritual practices help you develop a sense of inner peace and resilience. You start to see life from a more balanced, holistic perspective rather than getting caught up in the hustle and bustle. You gain a deeper understanding of yourself and the world around you, shaping your mindset in a more positive, healthy way.

So, while mindfulness and spirituality might seem like "new age" concepts, they're pretty grounded. They're all about finding what works for you and incorporating those practices into your everyday life. Because at the end of the day, your mind-

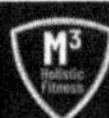

set is like a garden. You've got to water it, give it sunlight, and keep the weeds at bay for it to flourish. Mindfulness and spirituality? They're some of the best tools in your garden shed.

Finally, remember that practicing mindfulness and spirituality is less about reaching a specific destination and more about the journey. It's about developing a continuous practice, cultivating patience and compassion towards yourself, and embracing each day with a spirit of curiosity and openness. This journey is uniquely yours to explore, offering a pathway toward deeper self-awareness, inner peace, and holistic well-being.

Mindful Action

Imagine if every time you washed your hands, you could hit the reset button on your day. This simple act, which we usually do on autopilot, has the potential to become a powerful moment of mindfulness. When you engage fully, feeling the lather of the soap and the sensation of water flowing over your skin, you're not just cleaning your hands—you're grounding yourself, bringing peace and clarity into your day.

Think of it as more than just washing away dirt. Visualize all the stress, negativity, and distractions going down the drain with the soap suds. This mental imagery transforms an ordinary task into a powerful ritual, cleansing not just your hands but your mind and spirit. It's a quick, no-fuss way to reset your emotional state and regain your focus.

You don't need extra time or a special setup to make this happen. Just a shift in mindset can turn handwashing into a refreshing break for your well-being. These brief, intentional moments add up, helping you feel more centered and resilient throughout the day. So, next time you head to the sink, take those few seconds to practice mindfulness. You'll be amazed at the impact it can have, lifting your spirit and elevating your entire day.

ANCHOR 4 — CREATIVITY

Creativity isn't just a side dish in the grand meal of life; it's really the key to a full and authentic journey. Every time you grab a brush or a pen, you're not just making marks on a canvas or scribbling words on a page—you're actually letting bits of your soul spill out. This isn't just freeing; it's deeply therapeutic, providing a quiet mental space that can seriously dial down the stress. And it's all about the process and discovering new parts of yourself along the way.

If you're more inclined to write, then let those words pour out. It's not just about putting ink on paper—it's about penning what's bubbling up inside you. Whether it's journaling, tapping into some poetry, or stitching together a short story, writing can be like a mental detox, clearing out the old thoughts and making space for new insights and personal growth.

Creativity isn't just about traditional arts like painting or writing. Your kitchen and garden are canvases, too. Cooking turns you into a food wizard, blending flavors and textures into delightful creations that taste and feel good. Gardening is about tuning into the rhythms of nature, watching things grow and thrive under your care—a totally grounding and incredibly rewarding experience.

And for those of us who like to keep active, don't think creativity doesn't play a role. Have you ever thought about how dance is basically storytelling but with your body? How can you mix up your workouts with a little imaginative twist, turning them from mundane to fun? It's all about making each move count in a way that's enjoyable and personal.

Creativity really is a must for anyone looking to spice up their life—it's about making everyday activities a little more special and a lot more you. The M3 Method celebrates this, viewing creativity as a key pillar to living not just a good life

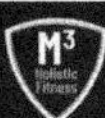

but a great one. It touches everything from how you think to how you feel and even how you move.

So, why not dive into something creative today? Paint, write, cook, or dance your way into a life that's not just lived but fully experienced. Embrace that creativity and watch how it transforms not just your moments but your entire life. You're not just crafting works of art; you're crafting a life that's rich, colorful, and deeply satisfying.

Spice Up Your Meals with a Creative Twist

Forget mealtime monotony; let's turn your kitchen into a canvas and your plate into a masterpiece! Imagine a 'Rainbow Dinner' that's more like an edible Pantone chart—splashes of red tomatoes, golden squash, verdant greens, and purples so deep they'd make a peacock jealous. This isn't just dinner; it's a full-on feast for the eyes and the soul. You're not just eating; you're savoring, discovering, and celebrating!

And the best part? Each color doesn't just brighten your plate; it supercharges your health with a spectrum of nutrients. Perfect for gay men over 50 who are looking not just to eat but to dine with flair and vitality. Now, who's ready to get cooking like Picasso?

Turn Your Workouts into a Creative Playground

Let's transform your workout into a playful experience! Picture this: every time you lace up those sneakers, you're stepping into a world of fun and creativity. Forget the mundane routine; let's make fitness something you look forward to!

Imagine turning your workout into a dance party with Zumba or hip-hop dance classes, where every move not only burns calories but also boosts your mood. Feel the music, let loose, and express yourself. It's not just about the steps or the rhythm; it's about enjoying the moment and feeling alive!

Have you ever considered blending martial arts with dance? Give Capoeira a try! It's not only a fantastic workout but also a powerful way to tell a story through movement. If you're a nature enthusiast, take your workout outdoors. Yoga on a serene lake or trail running through vibrant landscapes can turn exercise into an exploration of the natural world around you.

The key here is to find joy in the activity itself. Mix things up, challenge yourself with new and exciting forms of movement, and most importantly, have a blast doing it. With the M3 Method, it's all about bringing energy, joy, and a bit of playfulness to your fitness journey.

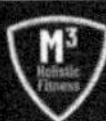

ANCHOR 5 — WORK-LIFE BALANCE

Finding the right mix between your work and personal life is a lot like maintaining a well-tuned orchestra—every instrument has its part to play, and the music only works when they all come together in harmony. Similarly, your life is a delicate composition of work, personal relationships, hobbies, relaxation, and self-care. They all need their moment in the spotlight to create a balanced and fulfilled life.

Let's start by considering the role of boundaries in achieving work-life balance. Establishing clear boundaries can be as simple as setting designated working hours and sticking to them or ensuring that your weekends are free for rest and relaxation. For instance, imagine you're someone who's been taking work calls well into your personal time. By setting a boundary, such as not accepting work calls after 6 p.m., you're carving out space for your personal life and setting a precedent that you respect your time.

Learning when to disconnect is another crucial aspect. In an era where you're always a notification away from work, knowing when to switch off your devices and engage in "screen-free" time can do wonders for your mental health. It could be designating the last hour before bed as a no-screen zone, where you read a book or have a conversation with a loved one instead. This not only helps you separate from work but also improves your sleep hygiene, leading to a more rested and refreshed mind.

Making self-care a priority is often overlooked, especially when deadlines loom and workloads pile up. However, it is in these high-pressure moments that self-care becomes even more critical. Self-care can take various forms; it could be physical activity, like a morning jog or yoga session, or more mindful practices like meditation. For instance, if you're a manager in a bustling firm, taking a 10-minute meditation break in your day can help you unwind, refocus, and handle stress more effectively.

Finally, it's important to remember that work is just one part of your life. Your personal life—including your relationships, hobbies, and leisure time—deserves just as much attention and care. Spending quality time with loved ones, pursuing a hobby, or simply taking a quiet moment to enjoy a cup of coffee can significantly contribute to your overall happiness and well-being. For example, if you're an entrepreneur who's always engrossed in business plans, dedicating time each week to a passion project like painting or hiking can provide a much-needed counterbalance and foster creativity.

In the M3 Method, finding work-life balance isn't just about splitting your time strictly but embracing flexibility and harmony among various aspects of your life. It involves recognizing the diverse dimensions of your life and nurturing each aspect—work, relationships, hobbies, and self-care—with the attention and room they deserve to thrive. Ultimately, a well-rounded life cultivates a positive mindset, paving the way to your happiest and healthiest self.

Balancing Work and Life for Your Mindset

Let's explore how this balance unfolds in the 'Mindset' component of the M3 Method. Imagine incorporating mindfulness into your workday—truly being present in each moment, aware of your thoughts and feelings, without judgment. This could involve taking short breaks ranging from 3 to 15 minutes to engage in deep breathing or meditation. These pauses serve as a much-needed buffer against work-related stress and pressure. Such mindfulness adds a layer of clarity, focus, and emotional equilibrium, making it a potent tool for maintaining a healthy mindset amid professional demands.

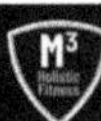

Balancing Work and Life Through Your Movement

In the 'Movement' segment of the M3 Method, work-life balance might entail scheduling regular workouts that don't get eclipsed by work obligations. Picture starting your day with a brisk walk or a swift workout before plunging into your tasks. Alternatively, you could schedule brief exercise breaks throughout the day for stretching or walking, breaking up the tedium of prolonged sitting. This regimen not only helps keep you fit but also reduces stress and enhances productivity.

Balancing Work and Life at Your Mealtimes

When it comes to 'Meals,' finding the right balance between work and life can be as simple as being present while you eat. We all know how crazy schedules can make us gobble down our food without really enjoying it. Picture this: setting aside specific moments for meals where work doesn't intrude. Just imagine having breakfast without checking emails or taking a real lunch break away from your workspace. Mindful eating allows you to savor every bite—its taste, feel, and aroma—helping you digest better and build a healthier connection with food.

Weaving Work-Life Balance into Your M3 Method

By weaving work-life balance into every aspect of the M3 Method, you pave the way for a harmonious and well-managed life filled with purpose and equilibrium. Whether you're practicing mindfulness to nurture a balanced mindset, savoring mindful eating for improved nutrition, or prioritizing regular exercise for fitness, these habits highlight the significance of balance in all areas of your life. This holistic approach helps ward off burnout and promotes general well-being so you can enjoy both your work and personal life to the fullest.

ANCHOR 6 — FINANCIAL FITNESS

Having control over your finances isn't just about filling your bank account to the brim; it's about clearly understanding your financial fitness and taking steps to maintain it. This awareness can be a catalyst for peace of mind and can reduce feelings of anxiety associated with financial uncertainties.

Setting realistic financial goals is a significant step toward financial security. For example, if you've always dreamed of taking a trip to Italy, don't just daydream—start planning. Break down the trip's costs into manageable savings goals that include airfare, accommodations, food, and sightseeing. Then, begin setting aside money each month. This approach not only instills a sense of purpose and direction in your financial journey but also introduces a habit of saving and planning that can benefit other areas of your life.

Thinking about your budget is important. When you plan and organize your finances, it helps pave the way for financial independence. By staying within your financial limits, you can easily steer clear of money worries. One useful approach is following the 50/30/20 rule: allocate 50% of your earnings for essentials, 30% for fun expenses, and save 20%.

Planning for unexpected financial situations is super important! It's a smart move to have an emergency fund that can ideally cover 5-6 months of living expenses. This fund can truly be a lifesaver in times of job loss or medical emergencies. For instance, if you're a freelancer with income that varies, having this financial safety net can bring you so much peace of mind.

Another consideration, especially for men over 50, is retirement planning. Even if retirement seems far away, starting early can help ensure a comfortable life later on. Simple steps like contributing to a retirement fund every month or investing in a pension plan can make a difference.

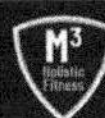

Understanding and managing debt is another part of maintaining financial fitness. If you have student loans, creating a plan to tackle them systematically can make the repayment process more manageable.

Lastly, financial fitness also involves regular check-ins on your financial health. Reviewing and adjusting your budget and goals periodically can keep you on track and help you adapt to changes in your life or income.

By following these steps, you'll feel less financial stress and open to a feeling of abundance. When money worries fade, you can dedicate more time to what truly brings joy to your life: connecting with loved ones, pursuing hobbies, and nurturing personal development. This feeling of security and abundance plays a key role in the M3 Method, supporting your mental and emotional wellness.

Finances and Mindset

It's important to begin by looking at how you think about money. When I was younger, I was always thinking in terms of scarcity, and this mindset stayed with me as I got older. The idea that there will never be enough, whether it's money, chances, or support, often brings about worry, stress, and making financial choices out of fear.

Recognizing this, I actively shifted my mindset and my relationship with money from one of lack to one of abundance. Think about it: it's easy to slip into a negative cycle, letting worry or a sense of scarcity cloud your judgment. This adds a layer of stress that's counterproductive to your overall well-being.

Imagine flipping the script. By embracing positive affirmations and visualization exercises, you can nurture a brighter perspective on money. These subtle yet powerful shifts in your mindset have the potential to positively impact how

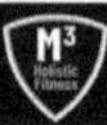

you approach and manage finances, guiding you towards improved financial well-being.

How does this relate to the financial well-being of men over 50? Moving away from a mindset of scarcity helps you embrace a more abundant outlook, which is key for making wiser financial decisions like saving, investing, and preparing for retirement. This strategy fits perfectly with the M3 Method's emphasis on achieving a sense of overall mental, emotional, and financial harmony. By letting go of scarcity thinking, you set yourself up for financial prosperity and a future filled with self-assurance and independence.

Finances and Movement

Staying fit can feel like it comes with a hefty price tag, with gym memberships and fitness classes. But there are plenty of ways to stay in shape without stretching your finances too thin. How about low-cost or free activities? Think running, walking, or working out at home. Or perhaps investing in a piece of workout equipment might make more sense in the long run compared to ongoing gym costs. These smart choices mean you can keep up your fitness without breaking the bank.

Finances and Meals

When you talk about meals, money comes into play. Eating a healthy diet doesn't have to break the bank. It's about making savvy choices that align with your financial goals. Take meal planning and prepping, for example; it's a time and money saver that prevents you from making impulse purchases and reduces food waste—great for your budget. Plus, cooking at home instead of dining out can be better for your wallet and your waistline. Use the concept of "cook once, eat twice." This involves preparing enough food at one time to generate two or more meals. These small strategies allow you to eat well without straining your finances.

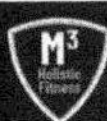

ANCHOR 7 — STRESS BUSTERS

Stress can be like a stubborn weight that you carry around, impacting both your mind and body. Just like how you work on building your muscles for strength and endurance, it's important to create methods that help you handle stress for your overall well-being. Think of it as a mental workout regimen: essential, empowering, and life- changing.

Stress often manifests in various ways, affecting your thoughts, feelings, and behaviors. Recognizing these signs is the first step towards managing it effectively. Examples of stress can include:

Emotional Symptoms: You might feel overwhelmed, anxious, or irritable. Persistent worry, mood swings, and feelings of sadness or depression are common indicators of emotional stress. Recognizing these feelings can help you understand that your mind is under strain and needs relief.

Physical Symptoms: Stress can take a toll on your body, leading to headaches, muscle tension, fatigue, and even chest pain. It might also manifest as digestive issues or changes in your appetite and sleep patterns. Pay attention to these physical signs; they are your body's way of signaling that it needs care.

Cognitive Symptoms: Stress can cloud your thinking and concentration, leading to memory problems and difficulty focusing on tasks. You might find yourself being more forgetful or struggling to make decisions. Recognizing these cognitive changes can prompt you to take steps to clear your mind and reduce stress.

Behavioral Symptoms: Changes in behavior, such as withdrawing from social activities, procrastinating, or neglecting responsibilities, can also indicate stress. You might notice an increase in unhealthy habits, like overeating, smoking, or drinking alcohol. Being aware of these behavioral shifts can help you address stress before it becomes overwhelming.

The key to handling stress lies in the word 'stress' itself. It's more than just a feeling; it's a handy acronym that guides you on managing stress well. When you incorporate these steps into your daily routine, you'll boost your resilience, enhance your mental well-being, and improve your overall health—similar to how a complete fitness regimen tones your body.

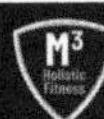

S.T.R.E.S.S.

S | Stop and ask if this stress is real: Before you let stress take hold, pause and assess the situation. Ask yourself if the stressor is genuine or if you might be overreacting or misinterpreting a situation. This self-reflection can help you gain perspective and prevent unnecessary stress.

T | Take time to breathe: When you're feeling stressed, your body's fight-or-flight response kicks in, which can lead to shallow breathing. Counteract this by consciously taking three deep breaths. Inhale slowly through your nose, filling your lungs, and then exhale through your mouth. This simple exercise can help calm your nervous system, reduce anxiety, and refocus your mind.

R | Respond, not react (or Rest): Instead of impulsively reacting to a stressful situation, take a moment to consider your response. This pause allows you to evaluate the best course of action, taking into account your feelings, values, and the potential consequences of your reaction. Alternatively, this step can serve as a reminder to rest, recognizing that sometimes a brief break is necessary to recharge and regain perspective.

E | Evaluate what you need: Take a moment to identify your needs in a given situation. Are you feeling overwhelmed, unsupported, or unprepared? By pinpointing your specific needs, you can begin to address them more effectively, ultimately reducing your stress levels.

S | Seek other options: Sometimes, the source of your stress is the belief that you have limited options or resources. Challenge this assumption by brainstorming alternative approaches or seeking support from others. Be proactive in communicating your needs and collaborating with those around you to find viable solutions.

S | Shift your relationship with stress: Changing your perspective on stress can be transformative. Embrace stress as a natural part of life and an opportunity for growth. Use the energy it generates to take positive action, whether that means resolving a conflict, seeking help, or adopting healthier habits. By embracing stress as an ally rather than an enemy, you'll be more equipped to cope with it and ultimately thrive.

Remember, the "STRESS" acronym is like a superpower in your stress-busting toolkit. Make these steps a habit to boost your strength and tackle whatever life throws at you.

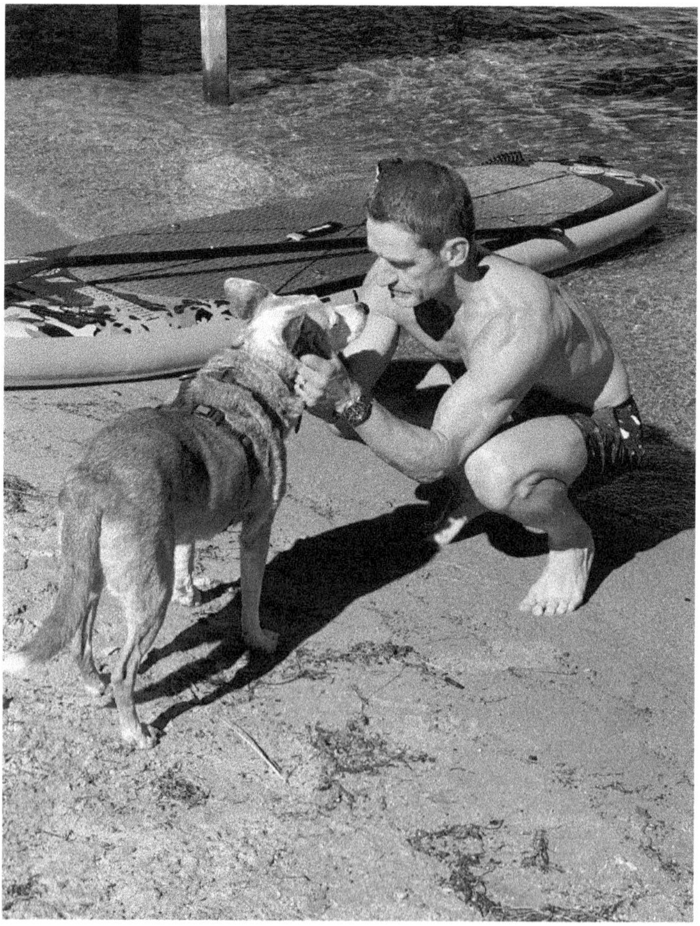

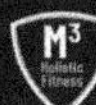

Mindset Actions

Review the following activities and complete at least three of them to help you integrate the Mindset content into your life. Bonus points if you accomplish all of them.

1. Reflective Journal Prompt: Today, identify one aspect of the M3 Mindset that resonates most with you. Write down three ways you can incorporate this into your daily routine.

2. Goal Setting Challenge: Set a small, achievable goal related to one of the M3 anchors. For example, plan a healthy meal or spend 10 minutes in mindful practice. Share your goal and progress on social media with a specific hashtag to create a community of support.

3. Mindset Shift Exercise: For the next week, start each day with a positive affirmation aligned with the M3 Mindset. Observe and journal about any changes in your mood or outlook.

4. Connect and Discuss: Check out our website for upcoming webinars, workshops and podcasts:

DirkSchultz.com

1. Creative Visualization Activity: Create a vision board that represents your ideal M3 holistic lifestyle. Use images and words that inspire you towards a healthier, more balanced life.

2. Weekly Challenge: Challenge yourself for one week to replace a negative mindset with a positive one in a specific area of your life. Note the changes in your journal.

3. M3 Method Workshop: Sign up for our interactive online workshop where you can dive deeper into each aspect

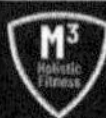

of the M3 Method and learn practical strategies to apply it in your daily life.

4. Daily Mindful Moments: Commit to spending 5 minutes each day in silent reflection or meditation, focusing on one of the M3 anchors.

5. Community Engagement: Volunteer or participate in a community event that aligns with the M3 Method. Share your experience and how it impacted your mindset.

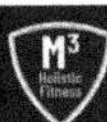

NOTES: WHAT DID YOU LEARN FROM THIS CHAPTER?

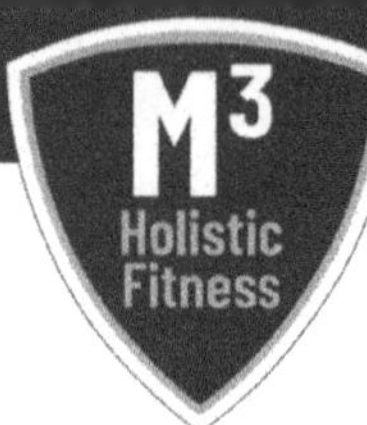

WHAT DOES YOUR LIFE LOOK LIKE?

1. Place a dot in each category to indicate your level of satisfaction with each area. A dot at the **center of the circle to indicate dissatisfaction** or towards the **outer edge to indicate satisfaction.** Most people fall somewhere in between. (see example)

2. Connect the dots to see your **M³ Circle of Life.**

3. Identify imbalances. Determine where to spend more time and energy to create balance. **This will help you create a better balance for your best Badass Life.**

SATISFACTION

DISSATISFACTION

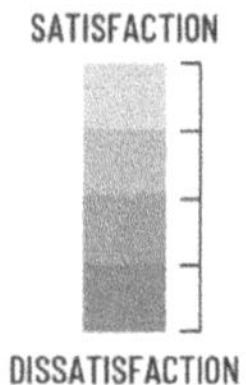

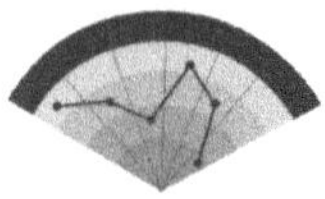

EXAMPLE

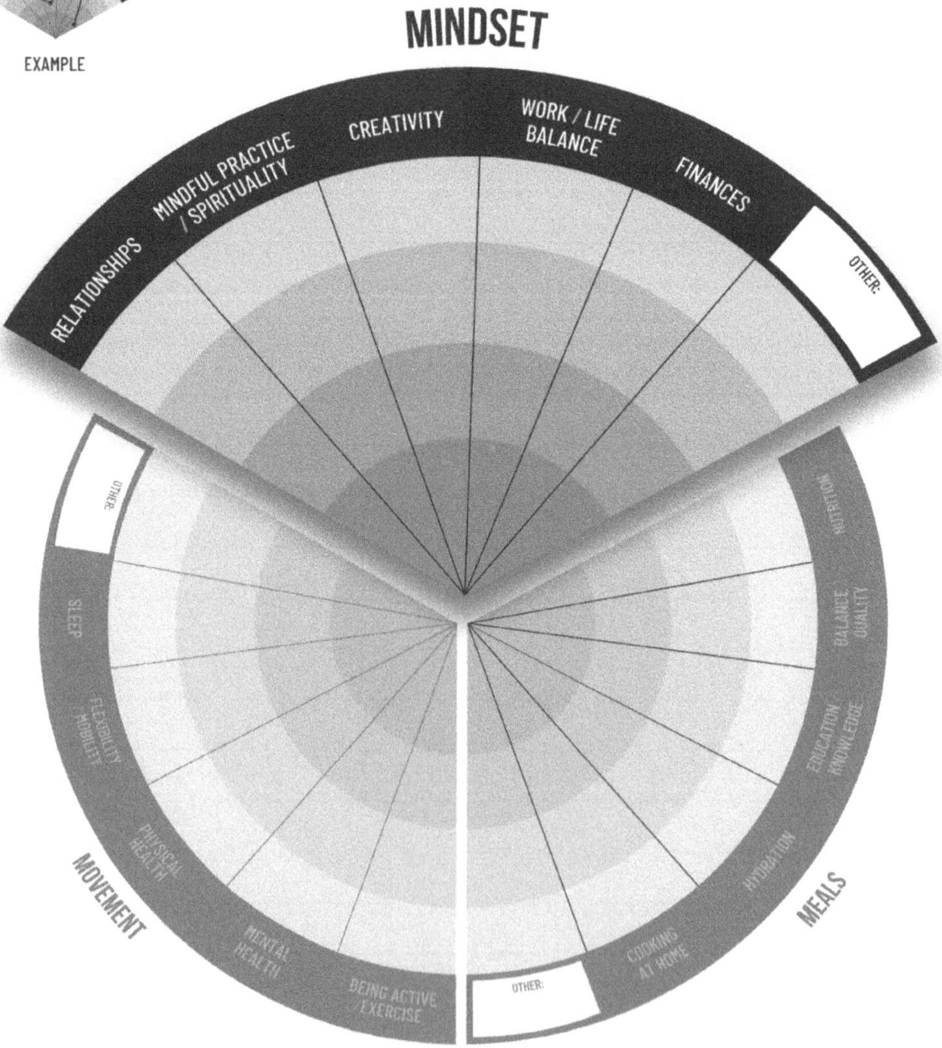

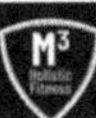

FREE DOWNLOAD

M3 Circle of Life Worksheet

http://dirkschultz.com/circle-of-life

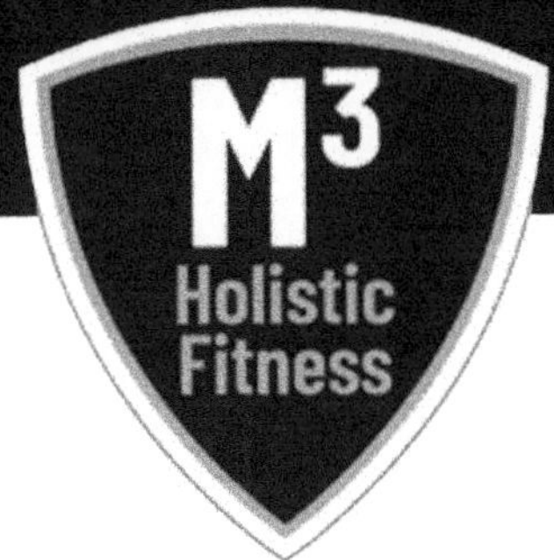

PART THREE

MOVEMENT

"Life is like riding a bicycle.
To keep your balance, you must keep moving."
— Albert Einstein

M·O·V·E·M·E·N·T

M | Mindful Momentum: Kickstart each activity with intention, using mindful momentum to elevate not just your physical movements, but also to activate positive change across all life's dimensions. See purposeful movement as your foundational springboard for holistic growth.

O | Optimize Wellness: Tune into your body to optimize movement for your holistic health. Whether you need rest, nourishment, or specific exercise, paying attention to your body's signals is key to maintaining well-being and preventing injuries or burnout.

V | Vary your movement: To cover all facets of your physical fitness, blend in cardio, strength, stability, and mobility exercises. Don't overlook the importance of rest days in your regimen. Vary your movement to keep both your body and mind actively engaged, adding a dash of spice to your routine.

E | Experiment and Embrace: Every step, stretch, and moment counts in holistic movement. Make workouts fun by embracing a playful, experimental spirit. Explore new activities that interest you while continually pushing for growth but remember to enjoy the journey.

M | Merge Mind and Body: Seek activities that integrate the mind and body, emphasizing their interconnectedness. Whether it's yoga, tai chi, or meditation in motion, find ways to unify these two aspects of self.

E | Energize Naturally: Harness the power of movement to invigorate both your body and spirit. Allow the natural energy boost from activity to replace artificial stimulants.

N — Nurture Through Movement: Use movement as a form of self-care. Just as you might nurture a plant by watering it, nurture your body and soul by giving it the gift of movement.

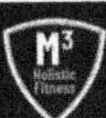

T — Thrive with Consistency: Recognize that consistent movement, even in small amounts, can lead to profound changes over time. It's about consistency and commitment.

This "MOVEMENT" acronym offers a comprehensive perspective on holistic health and the many ways movement can enhance your well-being.

Get off Your Ass!

Take care of your body.
It's the only place you have to live.
—Jim Rohn

If you're dreaming of a healthier, more vibrant life, it's time to embrace the simple, straightforward advice of the M3 Method:

"Get off your ass."

While the phrase might sound bombastic, the message couldn't be more important, especially as we age. Gone are the days when fitness was just for gym enthusiasts or yoga pros. In reality, the M3 Method is about integrating movement into every part of your day, from improving posture at your desk to enjoying a leisurely evening stroll.

With all the conveniences of mobile apps at our fingertips, they shouldn't replace the incredible energy and excitement that come from being physically active. We're designed to move, engage, and explore—not just to click and swipe. There was a time before smartphones when you had no choice but to move and be actively involved in your life, but now it has to be planned and intentional.

Let's break the habit of convenience and rediscover the fun in physical activity. It's not just about sculpting a great body; it's about being more physically involved in your life, connecting with yourself and your community more deeply, and truly engaging in all that life has to offer.

If you're dreaming of having that amazing life and ideal body you see when swiping social media, it won't just appear while you're binge-watching your favorite shows or endlessly scrolling. As we age, there is less time to achieve those benchmarks, and the benefits of staying active have become

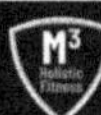

too significant to ignore. Sure, convenience is hardwired into our smartphones—food deliveries, rides with a tap—but this shouldn't overshadow the sheer importance of movement in your life.

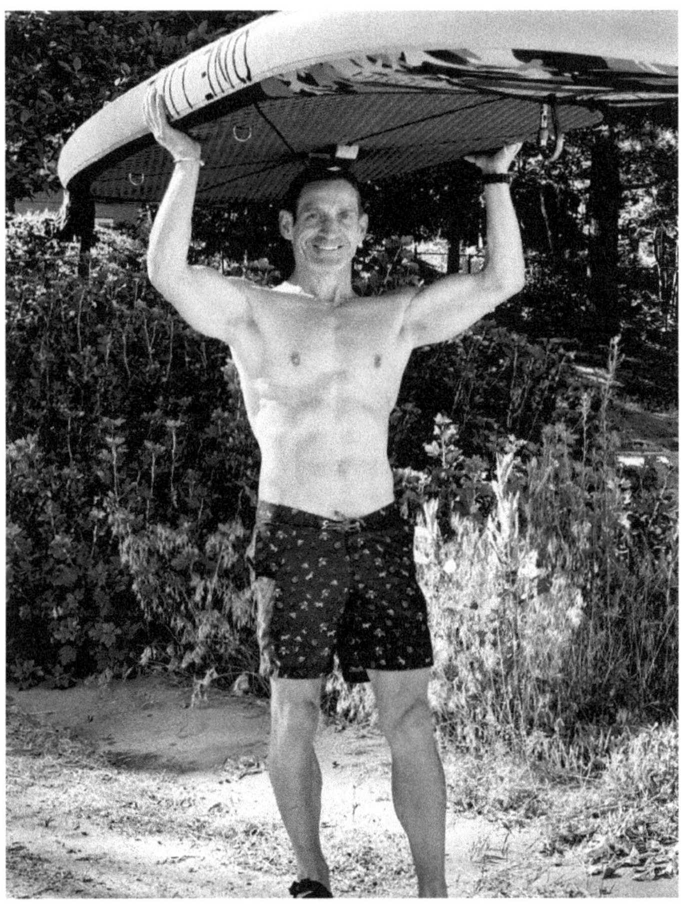

Let's rethink "movement" as something more than just sweating it out in the gym or perfecting a yoga pose. It's really about infusing harmony into your everyday life, connecting your body, mind, and spirit in everything you do. Whether it's sitting up straighter at your desk or taking a peaceful walk after dinner, movement is about being intentional and mindful of how you use your body throughout the day.

Movement benefits both the body and the mind. It can transform us by turning a bad day around into a time of reflection and insight. It shifts our mindset from the hectic "fight or flight" to a more serene "rest and digest," clearing our minds and serving as a natural antidote to stress.

Imagine you're having a rough day. Everything is going wrong, and stress is piling up. Instead of sitting around and dwelling on your problems, get up and go for a walk. Step outside, breathe in the fresh air and take in the beauty around you. Notice the flowers, the trees, and the sky. This simple act of movement can shift your focus from your worries to the incredible world around you, helping you feel better almost instantly.

Now, put aside the notion that only intense activities count as true exercise. Gentle movements like walking your dog, swaying to the music of your favorite song, or even moving busily around the kitchen are all meaningful movements.

In essence, movement is about embracing an active lifestyle that benefits not just the body but also the heart and mind. It's not about obsessing over metrics like steps or calories; it's about finding fulfillment with activities that resonate with you. Whether it's a scenic hike, a morning swim, or a round of golf, you're not just moving your body; you're recharging your mind and enriching your life.

If you're eager to fully embrace movement in life, why not explore the idea of having a coach by your side? A coach can design a customized plan that fits seamlessly into your routine, guiding you to reignite past interests or explore new ones. This way, staying active can be a source of daily joy. With their support, you can turn your health goals into tangible achievements and welcome a lively, enriching life.

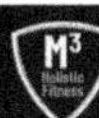

The Seven Avenues of Movement

Think of movement not just as a trip to the gym but as a multifaceted journey that touches every aspect of who you are. It's about integrating seven critical elements that collectively forge a fuller, healthier life.

Exercising and Being Active

Mental Fitness

Physical Wellness

Posture and Core

Mobility and Agility

Sleep Hygiene

And Yes — Sexual Fitness

Each plays a unique role in shaping your overall health. Whether it's the endorphins you get from a solid workout, the clarity you get from mindful meditation, or the rejuvenation you get from a good night's sleep, they all contribute to a more balanced you.

Let's not forget that staying limber and flexible ensures you can keep up with life's demands. So, when we talk about movement, it's about harmonizing these different areas to create a life that is bursting with energy, growth, purpose, and fulfillment.

Let's take a closer look at each of these six elements of movement.

EXERCISE AND BEING ACTIVE

Getting involved in the fun, challenging, and life-changing world of exercise is one of the most important steps toward health and longevity.

Whether you're in your prime years or just feeling prime, regular exercise is a game-changer. Think of it as your secret weapon for boosting energy, improving your health, and infusing your days with any adventure life throws your way.

While we can't sip from the mythical fountain of youth, lacing up those sneakers or unrolling a yoga mat and being active is as close as we can get to that magical elixir.

Regular physical activity slashes the risk of many age-related conditions and polishes our appearance to a more youthful sheen. More than just skin-deep vanity and aesthetics, physical activity translates into irresistible confidence and allure.

Who says sex appeal has an expiration date? Not us!

Adopting a lifestyle brimming with movement isn't just about physical health—it's a bold declaration of self-respect. It's a choice to strut through life with confidence, knowing that each step, stretch, or sprint is a statement to yourself and the world that you value your body and your life. Age really is just a number when you're jumping, jogging, or jazzercising your way through the best years of your life.

Now, imagine transforming everyday actions into fun and rewarding experiences.

Grocery Shopping as a Fitness Fiesta

Instead of viewing grocery shopping as just another chore, turn it into a mini fitness fiesta! Instead of parking near the entrance, choose a spot at the far end of the parking lot to get those extra steps in. As you navigate the aisles, treat your shopping cart like a dance partner: glide it smoothly as you lunge slightly to reach for items on lower shelves or do calf raises to grab the top shelf goodies. Each aisle offers a new beat to your shopping rhythm, making it a playful way to incorporate some light cardio and strength training into your

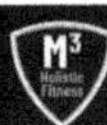

routine. End your shopping session with some bag lifting as you pack your car, enjoying the fun and active twist on a mundane task.

Cooking as a Calisthenics Kitchen Party

Transform your meal preparation into a calisthenics session to add a dash of excitement and movement to your cooking. While waiting for the water to boil or the oven to preheat, do countertop push-ups against the kitchen island or squats while stirring a pot. Incorporate calf raises while chopping vegetables or side lunges as you move from the fridge to the stove. Put on your favorite music to keep the energy up and dance around the kitchen between tasks. Not only does this make cooking more enjoyable, but it also turns meal prep into an opportunity for staying active, ensuring you're working on your fitness even while you cook up a storm.

Mall Walking: A Shopper's Cardio Circuit

Turn your next casual shopping trip into an invigorating mall walk with a dash of window-shopping cardio! Start by parking your car far away from the mall and walk to the entrance to get warmed up. Then, plan your route around the mall to include every floor and wing, transforming the enormous space into your personal walking track.

Challenge yourself to power walk between stores, pumping your arms for a heart rate boost. Incorporate mini lunges while browsing. Utilize escalators for calf toning by standing on tiptoes or climbing stairs two steps at a time for a more intense workout.

Incorporate flexibility exercises by reaching for the higher racks or squatting to sift through lower shelves. Treat yourself to dynamic stretches by reaching across clothing tables or twisting gently to grab items behind you. To keep things lively and engaging, make it a point to walk a lap of the mall before entering a new store, and at the end of your shopping session, cool down with a leisurely stroll and some window shopping. With each lap, you're not just browsing the latest trends but also boosting your stamina and energy, making your mall visit doubly productive.

Dog Walking with a Twist

Turn your dog into your cardio partner and transform your daily dog walk into a lively routine that's enjoyable for both you and your furry friend! Instead of the usual stroll, spice things up with a fun "obstacle course" approach to your route. Start by picking a path with varied terrain; think of a mix of grass, pavement, and sand if you're near a beach or park. This variety keeps the walk exciting and challenges different muscle groups for both of you.

As you walk, mix up your normal pace with short bursts of jogging or powerwalking, encouraging your dog to match your speed (safely, of course). Make use of park benches for light strength training like step-ups or tricep dips while your dog waits or sits by your side. If there are trees or lamp posts along your path, weave between them like a slalom ski course to improve agility and add a playful element to your walk.

Get creative with playtime during the walk: bring a ball or a frisbee for a quick game of fetch, which also adds sprinting intervals to your exercise. This not only increases your heart rate but keeps your dog excited and energetic about their walks.

By the end of your route, incorporate a cool-down period where you and your dog can slow down and enjoy a leisurely pace, helping to stretch out the muscles you've both used. This enhanced dog walking routine turns a daily chore into a fun and invigorating activity that boosts your fitness and deepens the bond with your pet.

As you can see, movement isn't just about maintaining fitness—it's about finding creative ways to enjoy what you are already doing every day.

So, instead of couch surfing, tapping, and scrolling, why not get off your ass, turn the music up, and let loose, turning everyday activities into your everywhere fitness routine. And remember to sneak in those quieter moments of movement for reflection and peace of mind—like a meditative walk through a lush park or a gentle stretching session under the open sky.

Here's the fix: moving our bodies is supposed to be a blast, not a chore. It's about choosing activities we enjoy and creating intentional movement in our everyday activities.

As we step into this journey of movement, we're not just ticking off fitness goals; we're creating a richer, more personalized life where the world is our gym and our playground. So, let's lace up, stretch out, and move like nobody's watching—because this vibrant, energetic life is all ours for the taking!

Let's make every move count towards a life that's not just lived but eagerly celebrated.

MENTAL FITNESS

Mental fitness is just as essential as physical health in achieving a holistic lifestyle. Think of it as a gym workout for your brain—it's not only about keeping your mind sharp but also about enriching your entire life. Regularly engaging in mental activities boosts decision-making, enhances emotional responses, and sparks creativity, leading to a richer, more engaging life.

Weave a variety of mental exercises into your daily routine. Dive into books that expand your understanding, participate in conversations that challenge your perspectives, and embrace new hobbies that stretch your cognitive limits. These activities are to your mind what weightlifting and cardio are to your body.

Staying mentally agile helps you make better choices by being more present in your life. Regular mental workouts help fortify your brain, enhance your mood, and contribute to emotional well-being, keeping you creatively vibrant.

Speaking of mood, mental activities have a way of triggering endorphin release, similar to the effect of certain antidepressants. Regular engagement in mind-challenging tasks can help stave off feelings of depression and anxiety, essentially serving as a mental health boost. Plus, who can overlook the value of self-reflection? Engaging in mindful activities broadens your perspective of life and opens the door to healthier lifestyle choices and new friendships and relationships. It's like a therapy session without the therapist.

But the perks of keeping your mind active don't stop at better mood and mental clarity. This practice also leads to improved physical recovery and greater overall well-being. Less stress translates to less downtime and more energy for enjoying life's little joys, be it a night out with friends, enjoying live music, or getting in that extra workout.

Just like physical exercise, mental activity can add years to your longevity. Keeping your brain active, fit, and engaged can help reduce the risk of age-related cognitive decline.

Mental fitness is not just about challenging your mind; it's about the quieter moments, too—like unrolling a yoga mat at sunrise, walking barefoot on a sandy beach, taking a brisk

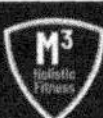

walk through your neighborhood, or choosing the stairs over the elevator. These simple choices are steps toward taking better care of yourself and cultivating the best version of yourself.

Mental fitness is easily overlooked, yet it is a fundamental component of the M3 Method. Committing to a mental fitness lifestyle helps keep your cognitive skills sharp, enhances your emotional well-being, contributes to your physical health, and may even add years to your life. It's the ultimate gift you can give to yourself because, with a clear mind, you make better choices for every area of your life.

Nature's Therapy

Nature is the ultimate elixir for every area of life and the perfect playground for getting off your ass and working on your mental fitness. Yes, you can have incredible body-only workouts while out in nature, but for most people, nature is the place they go to unwind and reset.

Consider quiet walks—where every step becomes a meditation and the surroundings a place of peace. The great outdoors offers more than just a scenic escape; it's a mental sanctuary. Here, you can unwind, let your thoughts wander, and reconnect with yourself.

These moments of solitude are not just calming—they're essential for mental clarity and self-reflection. There's something truly magical about feeling the earth beneath your feet, hearing the rustle of the leaves, and soaking in the beauty around you. Nothing quite matches the therapeutic benefits of being by yourself surrounded by life's natural beauty.

Whether in a peaceful park, a serene forest, or a brisk, breeze-filled beach, visit nature for peace of heart and mind. It is more than just a pretty backdrop; nature is the ultimate sanctuary for the soul. It's where you can reflect on your jour-

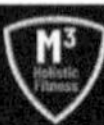

ney, recharge your spirits, and discover the inner silence to set new intentions for your life. These moments of solitude can soothe the mind and strengthen your sense of self.

Let's Get Social

Put that phone down and join a health club or community groups that offer more than fitness activities but are gateways to social activities and meeting new people.

You can level up your mental fitness by engaging in quality conversations, participating in book clubs, or attending seminars that keep your brain active and engaged. Get involved in community activities and events. Dust off that chess board and challenge a friend to some classic strategic thinking and problem-solving.

Get out of your comfort zone and enjoy a late night of Karaoke or go to a tea dance with your partner or friends. It's really quite simple. Get off your ass and create a rich life of socializing and lifelong learning. Mental fitness should be fun!

Wellness Treatments

Let's go to the spa! Wellness treatments like massage, acupuncture, and aromatherapy offer profound benefits that go far beyond physical relaxation and promote mental and emotional rejuvenation.

Regular massages are an important part of your mental fitness routine. By releasing muscle tension, your mental state also relaxes, providing a therapeutic escape that clears up your thinking and helps you make better choices.

Acupuncture, another valuable wellness treatment, can help manage stress and balance the body's energy flow. It's particularly effective in reducing anxiety and improving sleep, making it a powerful tool for mental clarity and stability.

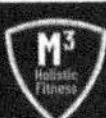

Aromatherapy uses essential oils to stimulate the senses and can significantly uplift mood and mental well-being. Incorporating aromatherapy into your routine can enhance focus, reduce anxiety, and promote a sense of peace and well-being.

By integrating these treatments into your regular self-care routines, you bolster your mental fitness, which is a fundamental value in living a full life with the M3 Method.

Expanding Your Mind

How about some mind expansion? Continuous learning is not just an activity; it's a lifestyle choice that plays a valuable role in maintaining mental fitness.

Make it a point to engage regularly in learning new skills and knowledge. This isn't just about gathering information—it's about challenging your understanding and expanding your perspectives, which keeps your cognitive abilities sharp and responsive.

Dive into learning a new language, mastering a musical instrument, exploring the art of cooking gourmet meals, or understanding the complexities of digital photography. Each new endeavor not only enriches your mind but also keeps your brain agile and ready to tackle new challenges.

Explore new books that provoke thought and stir curiosity helps you break away from familiar thought patterns and encourages mental flexibility. Audiobooks are a great way to learn new ideas and challenge your mind when sitting down with a book isn't feasible. You can listen to a book while driving, walking, running, cooking, or relaxing in a jacuzzi.

How about attending a live or virtual workshop or seminar that teaches you a new skill or introduces a business opportunity? These events not only present new ideas but also provide interactive experiences that exercise your critical thinking and problem-solving skills.

Every learning opportunity, whether it's reading a challenging piece of literature, participating in a lively seminar discussion, or exploring a new hobby, enriches your mind. By regularly engaging in new and diverse ideas, you continuously challenge and sharpen your mind and maintain your mental fitness.

The pursuit of lifelong learning is a cornerstone of the M3 Method. It enriches your life with continuous growth and development, ensuring you remain fully engaged and intellectually stimulated.

Exploring and Enjoying

It's time to break that routine, dive into new hobbies, and rekindle old passions. There's no better way to exercise your mind and enhance your quality of life than by injecting variety and newness into your daily routines.

Whether you embrace the creative flow of painting, master the culinary arts of cooking, take on a new sport, or write your first book, each activity stimulates different areas of your brain and expands your view of life.

Taking up photography, for instance, can sharpen your eye for detail and improve your appreciation of the environment around you. Gardening connects you with nature and can be deeply soothing, offering a sense of accomplishment as you nurture plants from seed to bloom.

These activities don't just pass the time; they enrich it. They provide opportunities for new areas of learning and growth. So, take the risk of getting out of your cocoon and exploring and enjoying new life experiences, discovering new ideas, and enriching your experience of life.

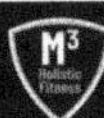

Building Community

There is nothing more important than a sense of community for gay men. Strong, supportive relationships do more than keep us company—they fend off loneliness and boost our mental fitness, turning our social networks into lifelines that give us a sense of connection and belonging.

In fact, the M3 Method sees community as the bedrock of overall health and wellness. Discovering and creating a sense of community with like-minded people who feed our souls is the very foundation of mental fitness.

Imagine joining a health club where the focus isn't just on physical fitness but also on developing real connections with people who share your interests and goals. It's not just about the workout; it's about the shared experiences, the mutual support, and the bonds we build while sweating it out or stretching in a yoga class.

Community is especially meaningful for gay men because so many of us do not have children or are outcasts from our families. Whether meeting up for coffee, attending a local event, participating in online groups, or planning holiday socials, every connection enriches our lives and strengthens our collective spirit.

Picture the fun and adventure of exploring new activities with friends, from weekend hikes to holiday parties that bring everyone together. And let's not forget the support we offer each other during difficult times, including the journey of coming out.

Having a strong community means knowing you've got people who understand and stand by you, ready to lift you up when you need it most. Having a supportive network can make all the difference.

With the M3 Community lighting the way, we can turn these connections into deep, lasting sources of mutual support, love, and friendship and help each other age gracefully with a smile on our face and a sense of belonging in our hearts.

Your Mental Support System

Have you ever noticed how the people you spend the most time with can influence your mood and outlook on life? It's true—your closest circle of friends and family can either lift you up or weigh you down. When it comes to mental fitness, the company we keep not only affects our mood but our attitude and choices.

We all have those friends or family we avoid because we know how they make us feel. Likewise, we also have those besties who we can count on for good vibes and happy times.

Think of each person in your life as a book in your mental library. Are they happy books or sad? Scary or uplifting? Inspiring or depressing? Do they add value to your life, or are they like those old magazines in a box in your closet or garage that get dusty and take up space? You know you need to let go of them, but you are still emotionally attached to those dusty old pages.

This is where the M3 Method steps in, reminding you to be mindful of who you surround yourself with. By removing negative influences and filling your life with positive and energizing people, you are essentially 'working out' your emotional and psychological muscles, strengthening your mental fitness just as you would your physical health.

It's about more than just having friends; it's about having the right friends. Those who challenge you, cheer for you, and cherish your every achievement. Like a gym buddy who pushes you to do one more rep, a good friend pushes you to grow, laugh, and thrive, even when life gets tough.

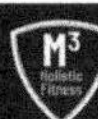

Furry Friends & Mental Fitness

Imagine this: you walk through your front door, and your dog's tail is wagging like crazy, or your cat is weaving through your legs, purring up a storm. If you've ever had a pet, you know that heartwarming feeling. It's like having your very own cheerleader waiting for you every time you come home. Pets are not just animals we share our space with; they're like furry bundles of joy that make our lives so much brighter. And for many of us, our pets are a key part of our mental fitness.

When you pet your dog or cat, it's more than just a touch; it's a moment of connection and caring. It's like they're giving you a big emotional hug. Petting them not only feels good but also has real benefits. It lowers the stress hormones in your body and boosts the feel-good chemicals. So, every cuddle with them is like getting a natural mood boost.

Having a pet also adds structure and meaning to your day. Feeding, grooming, and playing with them are not just chores; they're activities that give you something to look forward to. They give your day a purpose beyond what you do for yourself.

Plus, pets are great for making friends. Whether you're walking your dog in the park or chatting about your pet with a neighbor, they help you meet new people and make new connections. For the gay community, where many men haven't had children of their own, pets can fill that place of caring and nurturing.

Beyond just being fun, pets help keep us physically active. Regular walks and playtime are good for them and for us, combining exercise with the joy of being outdoors.

Pets also have this amazing ability to sense when we're feeling down and offer comfort without saying a word. They teach us empathy and how to care for others, which helps us take better care of ourselves.

Getting a pet means you're adding a special friend to your life, one that gives back so much love and loyalty. If you're thinking about getting a pet, remember that you're not just getting an animal; you're welcoming a new family member who will make your life richer and happier. They may be the very thing you need to elevate your mental fitness.

"There's No Place Like Home"

The place you call home is the most important part of your mental fitness. Do you feel at peace in your home, or is there chaos and tension? Your home environment sets the stage for how you feel about every area of your life.

In a perfect world, imagine stepping into your home and feeling a wave of peace wash over you. This isn't just any space; it's your place of retreat, perfectly curated to make you feel relaxed and at peace with yourself and life. But is it?

Have you ever noticed how a cluttered room can make your thoughts feel just as jumbled? Keeping your home tidy and free of unnecessary stuff is like giving your brain a breath of fresh air.

Every corner of your home can reflect and support your life's goals. From a peaceful corner perfect for meditation to an inspiring workspace that fuels your creativity, design each area with intention so that your home supports your bigger vision for your life.

The colors and decor you choose can influence your mood more than you might think. Choose soothing pastels or earth tones to create a tranquil vibe or brighten up your spaces with bold colors that energize and inspire. It's all about creating an environment that feels good to be in, one that lifts your spirits and sparks your creativity.

Think about how much smoother your day goes when everything you need is right where it should be. By organ-

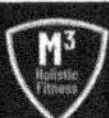

izing your home to keep clutter at bay, you're paving the way for less stress and more peace and productivity. Plus, there's nothing quite like the satisfaction of having a place for everything and everything in its place.

Make your home truly yours by decorating with items that hold important meaning or memories. A library with your favorite books, artwork that stirs the soul, or mementos from cherished travels can all serve as daily inspirations and reminders of what you love and where you've been.

A thoughtfully arranged home does more than just please the eye—it actively supports your mental well-being. Revamping your home to support your mental fitness isn't just a project; it's a transformation that parallels your growth. Each step you take to declutter and redesign not only enhances your space but also renews your mind.

Embrace this process and watch as your home—and your life—becomes a source of inspiration, peace, and rejuvenation.

Emotional Health

Emotional health and mental fitness go hand in hand. You can't have one without the other. To boost your emotional health, make sure you integrate self-care practices like Massage, Yoga, Pilates, Meditation, or Tai Chi. These will help you manage the stresses of life and relationships. This also means steering clear of people-pleasing behaviors, self-judgment, and being overly critical of others—these habits only add unnecessary stress to your life.

A good practice for emotional health is to set goals that are both achievable and believable. Small, realistic goals can create a sense of accomplishment and momentum. Finding your community is also important. Surround yourself with supportive people who lift you up and create a positive structure in your life.

Don't hesitate to seek professional help if you are continuously struggling with emotional health. A therapist can provide valuable guidance and support.

Remember, emotional health is a journey tied to mental fitness. It's about nurturing yourself, setting healthy boundaries, and prioritizing your well-being.

Life is Meant to be Enjoyed

Igniting your spirit is what mental fitness and living the M3 Method is all about—turning every day into a badass celebration of life. It's about more than maintaining physical health; it's about tapping into that deep well of joy and passion that makes life truly vibrant.

Start by connecting deeply with yourself. Find those activities that make your heart sing, and dive into them with wild abandon. Maybe it's embracing a new adventure, feeling the exhilaration with every fresh experience, or finding laughter in the little things that stitch your days together.

Living fully means savoring each moment and indulging in the sheer excitement of being alive.

PHYSICAL WELLNESS

It's easy to confuse physical wellness and physical fitness because they are similar but two different aspects of health.

Fitness is all about building up your cardiovascular, muscular, and skeletal systems with activities like cardio work-

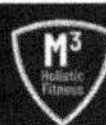

outs, strength training, and flexibility exercises to keep these systems in top shape.

Wellness is more about the overall healthy functioning of all your body systems as an integrated, holistic whole. This includes not only your physical health but also your emotional, mental, and social well-being, ensuring a harmonious balance that supports long-term vitality and quality of life.

Now, let's explore how this all plays out in your life, especially as you age. Aging gracefully isn't just about watching the years go by; it's about keeping our overall wellness in check by making healthy choices and steering away from toxic behaviors. Every stretch, every step, and every bit of activity we engage in is an investment in your longevity.

Here's how making a *physical wellness mindset* a regular part of your life can keep you thriving and looking your best.

Disease Prevention

There's a saying that goes, "An active body hosts a thriving spirit." And it's not just poetic; it's backed by science.

Engaging in regular physical activities, whether it's a brisk walk in the park or a weekly swim, provides a noticeable boost to cardiovascular health, keeps blood sugar levels in check, and strengthens bones. It's like giving your body a natural vaccine against a slew of health concerns. And in your vibrant 50s and beyond, this active shield keeps you thriving.

Physical Wellness Mindset

Let's dive into what it really means to adopt a physical wellness mindset. This isn't just about exercise; it's about choosing a lifestyle that elevates your overall quality of life every single day.

Step Up to an Active Lifestyle: Think of an active lifestyle as your secret ingredient for staying youthful and energetic. It's not about avoiding illness; it's about thriving. Regular activity boosts your immune system, keeps you energized, helps your skin look vibrant, and your body agile. Each step you take, each stretch you make, isn't just movement—it's an investment in your future self. Start simple: stretch each morning, take the stairs instead of the elevator, enjoy a morning stretch, and take those well-deserved walking breaks to invest in your future self. Small activities make a big difference.

Fuel Your Body: Let's talk about fueling that beautiful body of yours. Eating isn't just about satisfying hunger—it's about nourishing your body and mind with the best. Choose whole, unprocessed foods as much as possible—they're the premium fuel for your premium body. Drink plenty of water, eat vibrant fruits and vegetables, and watch how your energy levels soar.

Build Unshakeable Confidence: After a great workout, that glow you feel? That's confidence radiating from within. Physical activity doesn't just sculpt your body; it molds your self-esteem. Every push-up, every run, every swim builds not just muscle but a strong sense of "I can do this." Catching that smile in the mirror? That's you—powerful, confident, unstoppable.

Surround Yourself with Champions: Just as you nourish your body with quality food, enrich your life with quality people. Surround yourself with folks who lift you up and push you to be your best. These champions will make your wellness journey lighter and a lot more fun. Remember, we're social creatures, and the right crew can make all the difference.

Rethink Exercise as Your Power Outlet: Shift your view of exercise from a daily chore to your personal power outlet — an explosion of energy that keeps you feeling engaged

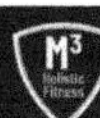

and spirited. Mix it up with activities you love—dance like nobody's watching, hike to see the sunrise, or play a sport that makes you laugh. Make moving a joy, not a job.

Embrace Emotional Wellness: This journey is as much about mental and emotional health as it is about physical fitness. Movement releases endorphins, our natural feel-good chemicals. So, when you exercise, you're not just strengthening your body—you're boosting your happiness and mental clarity.

Celebrate Every Step: Celebrate every bit of movement, every heartbeat, every breath. Each one is a victory, a moment of life fully lived. Join community groups, try new activities, and keep setting those wonderful goals. Every step is a step towards a more vibrant, fulfilling life.

POSTURE and CORE

Our parents and teachers were right when they said, "Stand up straight," so to speak. Proper posture and core stability are fundamental to keeping our back strong and healthy in and out of our workouts. How we set our posture and core before, during, and after a workout makes a big difference in the strength, durability, and longevity of a healthy core, back, and body. The power is in the posture.

Let's dive into why good posture matters so much. Proper posture is more than looking confident—it's the foundation for overall health and physical strength. When your spine is properly aligned, you reduce the risk of back pain and prevent wear and tear on your joints. Proper posture enhances breathing, boosts circulation, improves digestion, and keeps your energy levels high. It's not just physical health that benefits; standing tall can lift mood, boost confidence, and reduce stress.

We all fall into bad habits while sitting at a desk, driving, or even walking. But with some simple adjustments, you can correct that. Ensure your chair supports your lower back and your computer screen is at eye level while sitting. Adjust your seat so your back is straight, and your headrest supports your head while driving. When walking, imagine a string pulling you up from the top of your head, keeping your spine straight and your shoulders back. These small changes can make a big difference.

The Core Elements of Core Strength

A strong core is the foundation of good posture. Your core muscles support your spine, making it easier to maintain proper alignment throughout the day. A strong core improves balance and stability, reduces the risk of injuries, and enhances your performance in any physical activity. Plus, a strong core looks great and feels even better!

The 4-Step Posture Plan: Set. Brace. Align. Reset.

1. **Set Your Shoulders**: Roll your shoulders back and down. A tall posture not only looks good but also puts you in a position of power, ready to handle anything. "Shoulder back and down, as if you're putting them in your back pockets."

2. **Brace Your Core**: Imagine someone is about to tickle you. Engage your core just enough to create slight tension—not too tight. This small adjustment stabilizes your lower back and protects it from strain.

3. **Align Your Body**: Make sure your ears, shoulders, and hips are lined up properly for whatever activity you're

 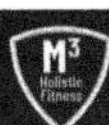

doing. Proper alignment boosts your performance and keeps your body moving efficiently and safely.

4. **Reset as Needed**: If you feel your posture slipping, take a moment to reset. This quick adjustment strengthens your form and signals your body that this is the posture you want to maintain.

The Power of Everyday Posture

Good posture isn't just for the gym; it's for every part of your life. Whether you're sitting at your desk, walking to your car, or relaxing at home, standing tall and proud helps you feel stronger and more confident.

Incorporate Mobility and Strength Training

To truly master your posture, add mobility workouts like yoga and Pilates to your routine. These practices enhance flexibility, balance, and core strength—all crucial for maintaining good posture. Pair them with strength training exercises like rows, planks, and squats to build the muscle support needed for a solid, upright stance.

A Final Thought

Standing tall and proud isn't just about looking good—though that's a great bonus. It's about feeling powerful, confident, and ready to take on whatever comes your way. Embrace the power of posture and watch how it transforms your strength, your health, and your life. So, let's make it happen. Every time you set, brace, align, and reset, you're telling your body, "This is how we stand; this is how we move, and this is how we conquer!"

MOBILITY and AGILITY

As you glide through your 50s, it's all about adding life to your years, not just years to your life. Flexibility and mobility are your secret weapons for living fully and freely. Staying bendy and spry allows you to stay active and zip through life's many detours and adventures.

To keep things smooth and spirited, integrating fun, flexible routines like yoga stretches, Pilates, Tai Chi, or dance classes into your daily schedule keeps those hips moving. These activities are not just good for your body; they're a blast and keep you feeling young at heart. Plus, keeping your muscles and joints limber helps dodge those pesky injuries that can slow you down. Think of it as greasing the hinges so the door to new adventures always swings wide open.

This focus on mobility means you can keep doing the things you love without a hitch, giving you the freedom to explore, engage, and enjoy every moment to its fullest. It's about making sure your golden years are golden in every sense—sparkling with activity, laughter, and plenty of motion. So, let's stretch, bend, and keep moving toward a future where every day is filled with potential and freedom!

The Power of Yoga

Yoga isn't just for the super flexible or the ultra-calm; it's for everyone looking to stretch a little deeper and breathe a little easier.

It's not about achieving complex poses but connecting with ourselves. Each stretch, breath, and posture offer both mental peace and physical flexibility.

 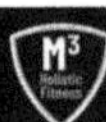

Stepping onto a yoga mat could mean stepping into a new phase of vitality and wisdom. Don't worry if you can't touch your toes on day one—yoga is more about the journey than the destination. It's about finding your flow and enjoying each moment of peace and stretching as your joints thank you and your stress levels drop.

Practicing yoga regularly will help you maintain joint health, improve your balance, and enhance your muscle strength. Plus, it's a great way to reduce stress and promote overall well-being.

When you step on a yoga mat for the first time, don't compare yourself to others. Instead, as you feel the tension, squeaks, and burning pain, don't think about how tight you are. Instead, say to yourself:

"Wow, this is exciting. I have so much flexibility to gain."

Yoga is not about losing tightness but gaining mobility and flexibility.

Benefits of Pilates

Pilates is all about control and core strength, but don't let that scare you away. It's not just for the fitness buffs; it's a gentle yet effective way to sculpt your body, enhance your posture, and move with ease.

Starting Pilates can feel like learning a new language of movement, but each session brings you closer to moving gracefully and living comfortably. Pilates can also help you improve your spinal alignment and build endurance, making everyday activities easier and more enjoyable.

Dynamic Stretching

Dynamic stretching is where Jazzercise meets Yoga and Pilates, blending the high-energy dance moves of Judi Sheppard Missett with the controlled, fluid motions of more traditional practices.

Picture yourself in your living room, outside on the grass, or at the gym; the upbeat music invites you to flow from one move to another. It's not just stretching; it's an energetic prelude to your workout or day. You might start with leg swings, each one like a dance step, sending vitality coursing through your hips and legs. Then, transition to arm circles that slowly grow larger, echoing the expansive movements of a dancer, opening up your chest and shoulders and setting a rhythm that your heart happily follows.

Incorporate walking lunges that propel you forward, each stride a deliberate move in your routine, echoing the functional grace of Pilates. Add in torso twists, a gesture that not only prepares your spine for movement but engages your core, echoing the mindfulness of Yoga with the dynamic twist of a dance routine. Finish with high knees, which could easily be a part of a high-energy Jazzercise class, pumping up your heart rate while preparing your legs for the activities ahead. This approach to dynamic stretching makes warming up a vibrant and essential part of your fitness regimen, infusing traditional flexibility exercises with the spirited fun of a dance class.

Balance Drills

Spice up your day with some balance drills that are not just functional—they're fun! As we get older, staying steady on our feet is key, but who says it can't be enjoyable? Try standing on one leg while brushing your teeth, walk heel-to-toe down a hallway as if you're on a tightrope, or challenge yourself on a balance board.

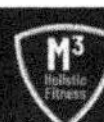

These simple activities pack a mighty punch, strengthening your core and leg muscles, boosting your coordination, and supercharging your confidence for all daily adventures. So, let's balance our way to a more stable and lively day!

Mobility and Flexibility

Keeping up the pep in your step as you age isn't just about the occasional jog or yoga session—it's about integrating mobility exercises that target key areas of your body to maintain youthfulness and energy. Let's explore some effective routines that focus on essential mobility zones: hips, spine, and neck.

Foam Rollers: Start with the all-star of self-care: foam rolling. Imagine this as a deep tissue massage you can administer yourself, ideal for soothing tight muscles around your legs, hips, and lower back. Regularly rolling out these areas can help alleviate stiffness and maintain your hip flexibility, which is crucial for everything from walking to maintaining balance.

Spine: For spinal health, incorporate yoga poses into your routine, such as the cat-cow stretch. This gentle flow, where you alternate between arching and rounding your back, isn't just soothing—it actively promotes spinal flexibility and strengthens the core muscles that protect and stabilize your spine. This is essential for maintaining posture and preventing back pain.

Neck: Don't neglect your neck—a region often strained by daily activities like driving or computer work. Simple neck rotations and tilts can greatly enhance the range of motion and relieve tension. Just a few minutes a day can contribute to better neck mobility and overall comfort.

Hips & Legs: Expand your routine to include hip circles and leg swings to target your pelvic area. Standing next to a chair for support, rotate your hips in large, smooth circles, then switch to leg swings. These movements not only lubricate your hip joints but also fire up the muscles in your legs and core, reinforcing balance and coordination.

By focusing on these key areas—hips, spine, and neck—and integrating these and other exercises into your daily life, you will enjoy the benefits of a body that moves as youthfully as you feel, keeping you active, energetic, and ready for life's adventures.

Embracing a Holistic Approach

Movement as we age isn't just about staying active—it's about committing to a lifestyle that fills every day with energy and purpose. This is at the heart of the M3 Method, which views movement as a key to unlocking a richer, more fulfilling life even as the years advance.

Imagine starting your day with a stretch that isn't just boring and static but a full, welcoming embrace of the morning. Each Pilates pose or yoga session becomes more than exercise; they are your personal moments of Zen that stretch your body and your potential. As you roll out a foam roller, you're not just easing muscle tension—you're rolling out the red carpet for improved mobility from your neck down to your hips and spine.

The M3 Method elevates this holistic approach by weaving these practices into a supportive community. It's all about connecting with others who share your journey and turning individual workouts into opportunities for deep, meaningful interactions. Within this community, movement evolves from a solitary activity into a shared adventure, enriching your experience and creating bonds that make every step more rewarding.

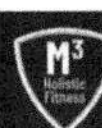

So, let's not just move to keep up; let's move to keep engaged. Dive into movement not just to maintain health but to enhance your vibrancy and enthusiasm for life. By engaging with the M3 Method, you're not just committing to physical activity—you're committing to a lifestyle that keeps you feeling alive, connected, and in tune with every vibrant moment life has to offer.

SLEEP HYGIENE

Let's talk about something that affects us all — sleep.

Sleep isn't just a nightly necessity; it's the unsung hero of our well-being, seamlessly intertwining with every facet of our lives. From sharpening our minds to healing our bodies, the quality of our sleep can be the difference between feeling like a champ or like we're running on empty. And let's face it, a good night's sleep makes everything better—our mood brightens, our energy levels soar, and even our minds and decisions get a little sharper and wiser.

However, for many, especially as we age, getting those blissful ZZ's can feel like a nightly battle with insomnia, sleep apnea, or restless legs syndrome. These are not just minor annoyances; they're like thieves in the night, stealing our rest and, with it, our zest for life. They leave us dragging through the day, sap our productivity, and, over time, can lead to more sinister health woes like heart disease and diabetes.

But here's the good news: You're not doomed to toss and turn into oblivion. There are concrete steps you can take to turn your sleep from frustrating to rejuvenating.

Developing good sleep hygiene isn't just about catching more hours of shut eye; it's about enhancing the quality of each hour. Simple adjustments to your bedtime routine, like setting a consistent sleep schedule, creating a restful environment, and winding down with a pre-sleep ritual, work wonders.

By prioritizing good sleep hygiene, you're not just investing in better nights; you're setting yourself up for more vibrant days. Imagine waking up not just feeling okay but feeling fantastic and ready to take on the world. That's the power of restorative sleep, and it's within your grasp. Let's commit to making those restful nights a non-negotiable part of our lives, ensuring we all wake up to days filled with energy and enthusiasm. Let's make sleep our secret weapon for a thriving, vibrant life.

Consistent restful sleep is so important it deserves its own acronym.

S —Set Up a Relaxing Environment

L—Leave Your Worries Behind

E—Eat Earlier

E—Exercise Wisely

P—Power Down Electronics

S | Set Up a Relaxing Environment: Creating a comfortable sleep environment is essential to getting a good night's rest. The bedroom should be quiet, dark, and cool. Heavy curtains or blinds can block out light, earplugs or white noise machines can block out noise, and a fan or air conditioner can maintain a comfortable temperature. Additionally, establishing a bedtime routine can help set your body's internal clock, and it can include activities such as taking a warm bath, reading a book, or practicing relaxation techniques.

L | Leave Your Worries Behind: Leaving your worries outside the bedroom is important to ensure a restful night's sleep. Doing a mind dump before bed can help free up space in

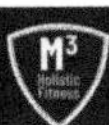

your mind, making it easier to relax and fall asleep. Write out any worries or concerns in a journal or on a piece of paper. It's also essential to avoid heavy conversations and watching the news before bed, as they can increase stress levels and make it harder to fall asleep.

E | Eat Earlier: Eating a large or spicy meal before bed can cause discomfort and indigestion, making it difficult to fall asleep. Eating at least two hours before bedtime is important to allow enough time for digestion. Additionally, it's best to avoid alcohol and caffeine for at least three hours before bed, as they can interfere with sleep quality.

E | Exercise Wisely: Exercise is beneficial for overall health and can improve sleep quality. However, exercising at least three hours before bed is best to allow enough time for the body to cool down. Working out later in the evening can increase alertness and make relaxing and falling asleep harder.

P—Power Down Electronics: Blue light emitted by electronic devices such as smartphones, tablets, and laptops can suppress the production of melatonin, a hormone that regulates sleep-wake cycles. It's crucial to power down all electronics at least 30—60 minutes before bed to allow the body to prepare for sleep. This can be achieved by setting boundaries for screen time and creating a relaxing bedtime routine that doesn't involve electronics.

Benefits of Good Sleep Hygiene

Improved Mood: Quality sleep helps regulate emotions and can reduce the risk of mood disorders such as depression and anxiety.

Enhanced Cognitive Function: Adequate sleep improves concentration, memory, and problem-solving skills, helping you perform better at work and in daily activities.

Better Physical Health: Consistent restful sleep supports immune function, reduces inflammation, and lowers the risk of chronic conditions such as heart disease, diabetes, and obesity.

Increased Energy Levels: Quality sleep helps you feel more refreshed and energized throughout the day, allowing you to engage in physical activities and maintain a healthy lifestyle.

Weight Management: Sleep plays a role in regulating hormones that control hunger and appetite, which can aid in maintaining a healthy weight.

Following the "SLEEP" acronym can help establish healthy sleep habits and improve the quality of your sleep. Creating a comfortable sleep environment, leaving your worries outside the bedroom, eating earlier, exercising wisely, and powering down electronics are all essential elements of good sleep hygiene. By adopting these habits, you can enjoy restful, rejuvenating sleep and wake up feeling refreshed and ready to tackle the day ahead.

Addressing Sleep Disorders: If you continue to struggle with sleep despite practicing good sleep hygiene, it might be time to consult a healthcare professional. Conditions like insomnia, sleep apnea, and restless leg syndrome can significantly impact your sleep quality and overall health. A healthcare provider can help diagnose these issues and recommend appropriate treatments or therapies.

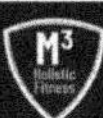

SEXUAL FITNESS

Take it from the "Top!"

Sexual fitness and holistic health are not reserved for the sprightly and spry; for many 50+ gay men, this golden era can spark a sexual renaissance—teeming with exploration, bursting with newfound confidence, and rich with satisfying encounters.

Let's be clear: sexuality isn't all we are, but it's an exhilarating part of our essence. As the years accumulate, there's absolutely no reason to shelve feelings of desirability, vitality, or pride in your physique.

Enter the M3 Method, your ticket to bringing sexual vitality into sharp focus and a reminder that age should never be a barrier to a rich, spicy sex life. It's about flipping the script on societal norms, demonstrating that life on the 5th floor can indeed be the most sexually charged and empowering years of your life.

Central to thriving in sexual fitness is mindset because your self-perception shapes every sexy encounter. It's time to strip away the doubts dressed up by ageist stereotypes and slip into the freedom that maturity offers. This isn't just a physical regimen; it's accepting where you are right now, honoring your desires without a hint of judgment, and approaching your sexual escapades with curiosity and an open heart.

Consider your mind as your largest erogenous zone. If we let it be overrun by negative chatter, we miss the thrill of the present moment. The M3 Method steers you towards developing a playful, positive mindset that can transform everyday interactions into peak "OH HELL YEAH!" moments.

Incorporate regular physical activities that amplify your strength, stamina, and flexibility, and you're not just caring for your heart—you're jazzing up your sex life. By nurturing emotional connections and fortifying mental well-being, you lay the groundwork for deeper, more satisfying encounters that rejuvenate your entire self.

So, put on your party best and watch as every slice of your life, including your sexual verve, sizzles with renewed vigor and delight. This journey isn't about chasing lost youth; it's about reveling in the sophisticated, sexy confidence that only comes with rich life experience. Let's break those molds and flaunt just how vibrant and sultry 50+ can be!

Movement and Sexual Fitness

When it comes to Movement, age is just a number. You may not be as nimble as you were at 20, but that doesn't mean your sexual vitality or body confidence is on a downturn. Exercise plays a key role in maintaining and enhancing your sexual fitness. It's not just about physical performance; it's also about feeling good in your own skin, boosting your self-esteem, and, let's face it, looking good naked.

Why is exercise so critical in this equation? It's more than just the immediate advantages like increased stamina or a stronger physique; it's about the long-term benefits that spill over into every area of your life, including your sexual well-being. Regular exercise not only helps you maintain a healthy weight, which is crucial for hormonal balance, but it also improves your cardiovascular health. Good blood circulation is a key component for sexual function, ensuring all your bits and pieces are working as they should.

Exercise also releases endorphins, the feel-good hormones that can boost your mood and alleviate stress, allowing for more mental space to focus on sexual pleasure. Feeling good in your skin enhances your self-confidence, something

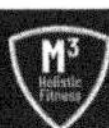

that doesn't go unnoticed in intimate moments. And let's not underestimate the sheer physicality of sex; it's an activity that can be both enjoyable and physically demanding. Having a strong, flexible body means you can adapt to different positions, rhythms, and scenarios as the moment moves you.

Beyond just performance and pleasure, exercise allows you to remain engaged in your own life, anchoring you in a sense of bodily autonomy that becomes a wellspring for sexual vitality and overall happiness.

Here's your sizzling lineup of exercises that will boost your sex appeal and pump up your mojo. Each move not only primes your body for peak performance but also adds a dash of excitement to your fitness routine:

Yoga: Unleash the power of flexibility and mental clarity with yoga. This isn't just stretching—it's about tuning into your body's whispers and turning them into roars of pleasure. Perfect for those who want to enhance their sensitivity and awareness, yoga makes every touch and sensation more intense.

Hip Thrusts: Get ready to turbocharge your hips and glutes with hip thrusts. These are not just exercises; they're tickets to stronger and more confident movements in the bedroom. Essential for boosting your performance and durability during those intimate moments.

Kegel Exercises: Who said Kegels are only for new moms? Men, get in on this secret, too. Strengthen your pelvic floor muscles for improved control and earth-shaking orgasms. It's a discreet workout with deliciously private rewards.

Bridges: Elevate your bedroom game with bridges. By targeting the glutes and pelvic area, bridges enhance your thrusting power, ensuring that every move is as strong as it is smooth. Feel the burn and enjoy the returns.

Push-ups: Build endurance and arm strength with the good old push-ups. They are ideal for sustaining those adventurous positions longer without a wobble: the more push-ups, the more possibilities in your love playbook.

Planks: Core strength is sexy, and planks are here to prove it. Stabilize your entire body, making those dynamic and challenging positions feel like a breeze. It's about holding on just as much as it is about letting go.

Cardio: Any form of cardio can boost your heart health and endurance. Run, swim, or walk your way to a more vigorous heart and lungs. You'll not only keep up without getting winded, but you'll also have the energy to go all night long.

Stretching: Become a master of motion with regular stretching. Enhancing your flexibility allows for creativity in the bedroom—because variety is the spice of life, and flexibility lets you enjoy all the flavors.

Squats: Build those legs for power with squats. This foundational exercise improves your lower body strength, which is critical for many sexual positions, and adds that extra oomph when it matters most.

Lunges: For fluid and graceful movements, integrate lunges into your routine. They enhance the strength and flexibility of your legs and hips, ensuring that your motions are both controlled and passionate.

Interval Training (HIIT): Short on time but high on desires? HIIT packs a punch by improving stamina and burning fat fast. These quick bursts of intense activity followed by rest will keep you dynamic and ready for action.

Sprinkle these exercises throughout your week and watch as your body transforms into a more powerful, confident, and

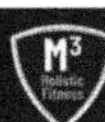

sexually vibrant version of yourself. Here's to a healthier, happier, and more thrilling bedroom adventure!

Meals and Sexual Fitness

Let's spice up the conversation about meals and sexual fitness. It's not just about the hearty dishes on your plate but also the vitality in your everyday life. Think of your meals as a direct feed to your sexual energy, especially pivotal for men over 50, where every bite counts not just for your taste buds but for your overall mojo.

On the menu for maintaining your sexual vigor, start with foods that do more than satisfy hunger. For instance, black raspberries and pine nuts are not just snacks; they're secret weapons for boosting libido and stamina. Avocados? They're packed with heart-healthy fats and vital B6, fueling both your heart and your heat. And let's not overlook the surprising perks of watermelon and olive oil, which enhance blood flow so effectively you might sideline those blue pills. Broccoli might be the unsung hero here, subtly boosting testosterone levels and keeping your libido in check.

Now, what to avoid? It's wise to sidestep the passion killers like spicy foods that might upset your stomach, carbonated drinks that can make you feel bloated, and too much processed and refined sugar and alcohol, which can extinguish your inner fire. Also, be wary of refined carbs—those sneaky testosterone diminishers that can add pounds and shift your hormonal balance.

But the journey to enhanced sexual fitness isn't just about filling your plate with the right foods—it's also about managing your health holistically. Regular medical check-ups and hormone level assessments are crucial.

Stepping away from the table, let's dive into the intangible ingredients of sexual fitness. What's your vision for your intimate life? Reflecting on your sexual desires and setting clear goals can sharpen your focus. Communication is your golden tool here, both with your partners and within yourself. Understand and articulate your desires, boundaries, and dreams.

And finally, infuse playfulness into your approach. Doing so isn't just about pleasure; it's about bringing a sense of lightness and exploration that rejuvenates both you and your relationships. Being truly present in each moment enhances not just your sexual experiences but enriches your life with greater excitement and deeper connections. Let's make meals—and moments—matter in the delicious journey of life beyond 50.

Those Pesky Hormones

If your dietary adjustments are not sparking the change you were hoping for, it might be time to consider hormone replacement therapy. However, approach this option with care and informed consideration. Remember, the science behind our bodies is intricate. Regular blood tests to monitor hormone levels play an essential role in maintaining sexual fitness and overall well-being, particularly for men over 50. Hormonal imbalances can subtly influence everything from your energy to your libido. If natural adjustments fall short, discussing hormone replacement therapy with your healthcare provider could be the next step to recalibrating your body's needs.

The "Bottom" Line

As we cruise into and past our 50s it's time to dial up the heat on sexual fitness. Think of it as fine wine—only getting better with age. Your journey to peak sexual health is unique, filled with personal tweaks and flirtatious fun, ensuring that your golden years are not just golden but absolutely sizzling.

Incorporating the right mix of nutrition, emotional wellness, and a cheeky check-up of those hormone levels can make all the difference.

Sprinkle your diet with libido-loving foods like avocados and nuts, and cut back on passion killers like excessive sugar, alcohol, and spicy late-night snacks. Remember, it's about feeling good inside to shine on the outside.

And don't forget the power of laughter and connectivity in keeping things lively. A good giggle can be just as stimulating as any aphrodisiac. So, lace up those dancing shoes, embrace the journey with a playful spirit, and keep the bedroom antics adventurous and alive. Your sexual fitness isn't just a side note to your health—it's the spicy headline.

There once was a man named McGee,
Who was fit as a feller could be.
With a wink in his stride,
He'd more often confide,
"It's my nightly routine that's the key!"

He'd twirl and he'd whirl with such grace,
In the bedroom, a marvelous place.
With a laugh and a leap,
Rarely did he need sleep,
Proclaiming, "It's all in the chase!"

Sunrise to Sunset

Every morning, as the first light nudges you awake, you are handed a blank slate—a fresh chance to steer your day toward what truly matters. Imagine the dawn as your personal restart button; with each sunrise comes the promise of renewal and the freedom to shape your day with intent.

There is magic to morning rituals. Kicking off your day with purpose isn't just about getting up; it's about rising with clarity, energizing your senses, and embracing your full potential for a vibrant day ahead. Let's explore how shaping your mornings can transform not just your day but your entire life, from sunrise to sunset.

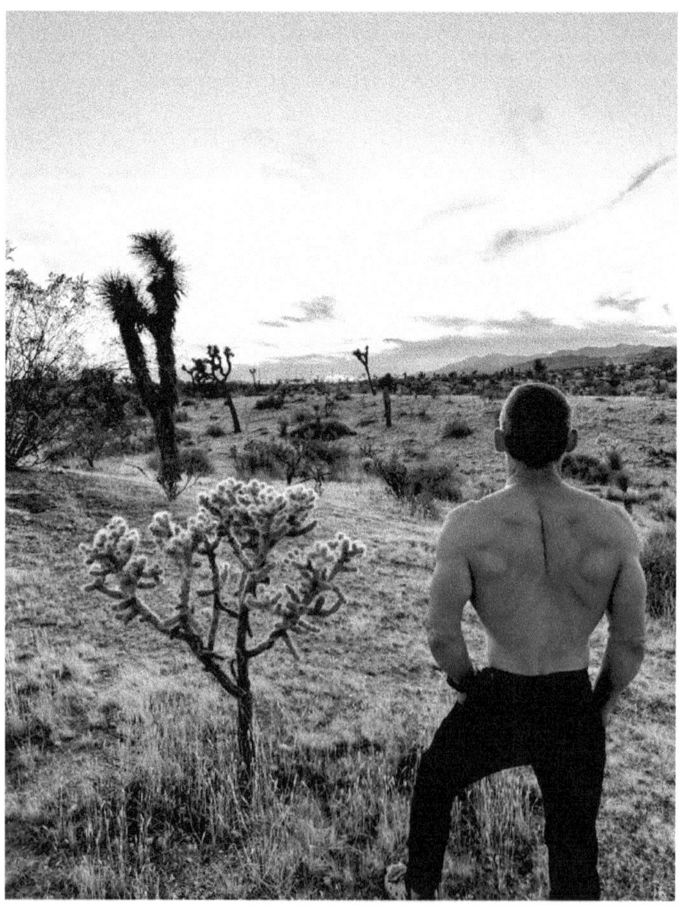

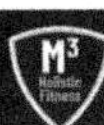

Picture this: Your day begins not with the jarring clamor of an alarm, but with a personalized routine that recharges your spirit, fuels your determination, and sharpens your focus. This isn't just about starting your day; it's about owning it. Your morning ritual sets the rhythm, creating a symphony of activities that nourish both body and mind—be it through rejuvenating exercise, serene meditation, or a moment of gratitude.

But how exactly do you craft a morning ritual that resonates with your personal needs and aspirations? It's about finding what invigorates you, what centers you, and what gives you a sense of purpose as you step into your day. Let's delve into how to establish these energizing routines and make them a steadfast part of your mornings, ensuring each day begins with momentum and meaning.

SUNRISE

Design Your Morning Ritual

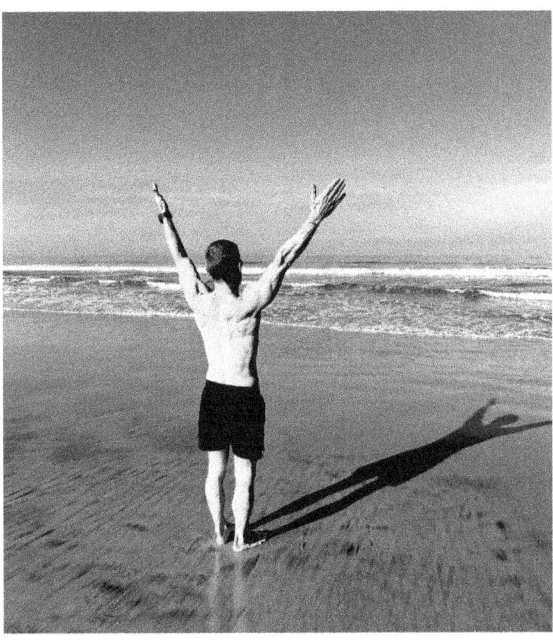

Rise and Align

Before your smartphone and the digital world start tugging at your attention, why not carve out a moment just for you?

Here's a tip to get you grounded, focused, and perfectly aligned for the day ahead: Kick off your morning with a large glass of water. It's simple but impactful. After a night of rest, your body is naturally dehydrated, and there's no better way to wake up your system than hydrating it thoroughly. This first step is like pressing the reset button, giving your body a clear signal that it's time to start anew. So, fill up that glass and make your first act of the day one that replenishes and refreshes.

Prioritize Physical Activity

Morning is an ideal time to engage your body and raise your energy levels. Whether it is a brisk walk in the cool morning air, a high—intensity interval training (HIIT) session, or a calming yoga routine, physical activity stimulates blood flow, enhances alertness, and contributes to overall health. Exercise also triggers the release of endorphins, the body's natural mood lifters, setting a positive tone for the rest of your day.

Embrace Mindfulness

Follow your physical activity with a mindfulness practice to ground you in the present moment. This can be meditation, journaling, or simply savoring a cup of tea in quiet contemplation. The key is to anchor your attention in the here and now, creating a tranquil space amid the noise of daily life.

Nourish Your Body

Breakfast has long been lauded as the most important meal of the day. Eating a balanced, nutritious breakfast fuels your body for the day's challenges and helps to regulate your

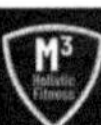

metabolism. Choose foods rich in protein, fiber, and healthy fats to support sustained energy levels and maintain satiety.

Set Intentional Goals

Before the day sweeps you up in its ebb and flow, take a moment to outline your objectives. What do you want to achieve today? Setting clear, achievable goals can channel your energy towards meaningful action. It also provides a sense of accomplishment when you tick off completed projects.

Focus on Gratitude

Beginning your day with a sense of gratitude can elevate your mood and broaden your perspective. A daily gratitude practice, such as writing down three things you're thankful for, can shift your focus from what's lacking in your life to what is abundant.

Remember, the most effective morning ritual is the one that resonates with you and complements your lifestyle. Be flexible and open to adjustments as you discover what practices serve you best. Your ritual may evolve with you, reflecting changes in your schedule, priorities, or wellness goals.

Also, don't pressure yourself to create an elaborate morning ritual overnight. Start small, perhaps with just one or two practices, and gradually incorporate more elements. Consistency, not complexity, is the key to a successful morning ritual.

A morning ritual is not merely a sequence of tasks but a harmonious symphony of habits that sing to the rhythm of your well-being. By choosing to rise and align each morning, you're not only investing in your health and fitness but also your growth as a person. Embrace the beauty of a purposeful morning and witness the profound impact it has on the trajectory of your day and, ultimately, your life.

SUNSET

Embrace the Night

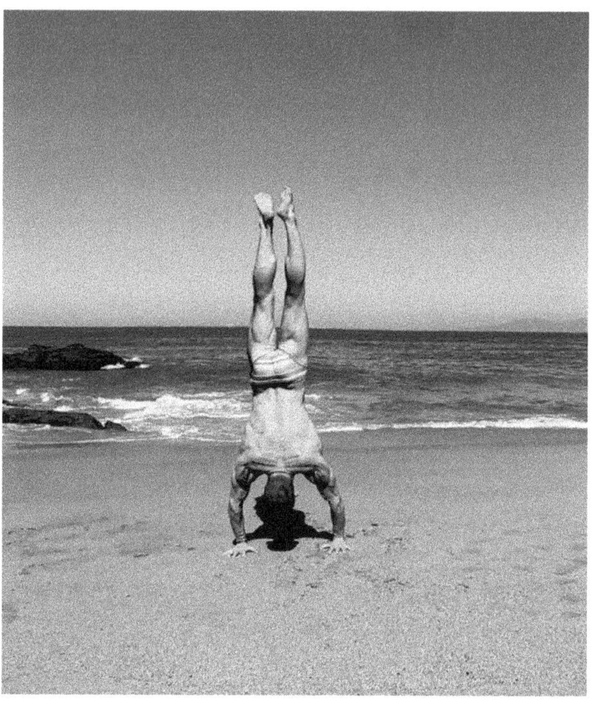

As the sun dips below the horizon and the world wraps itself in a gentle blanket of stars, it's time for your body and mind to begin winding down.

Just as the morning ritual sets the tone for the day, a purposefully crafted bedtime ritual can be the key to achieving restful and rejuvenating sleep, a foundation for good health and clarity. After all, our days are not just shaped by how we start them but also by how we choose to end them. Recognizing the importance of transitioning into night can be the secret to unlocking a holistic sense of well-being.

From gentle stretching to deep breathing exercises, each element serves as a token of self-love, building the bridge between an active day and a peaceful night. Consider in-

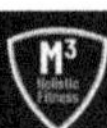

dulging in gentle yoga or Pilates, allowing the stretching to release any tension. Or spend some time with a foam roller, smoothing out any knots that the day may have tied.

Your Evening Night Cap

Your evening nightcap is more than just a winding-down routine; it's an essential ritual that balances your day and prepares you for what's ahead.

Start by letting go of physical tension through light stretching or yoga, embracing techniques like progressive muscle relaxation to give your body that "ahhh" moment. This physical release primes you for mental relaxation and paves the way for thoughtful introspection. Spend a few quiet moments reflecting on the day's highs and lows, perhaps jotting them down in a journal. This practice not only helps you process emotions but also serves as a springboard for setting tomorrow's intentions.

Now that you've stilled your body and examined your thoughts, it's time to nourish your mind. This could mean getting lost in the pages of a compelling novel, getting carried away by some soul-soothing music, or floating through a guided meditation. The aim here is to engage in activities that enrich your spirit without overstimulating your senses—think more along the lines of gentle, ambient sounds and less like the glare of a smartphone screen.

Once you're feeling relaxed and centered, take a moment to set yourself up for a smooth morning. Lay out tomorrow's outfit, arrange your essentials, or even draft a quick to-do list. The peace of mind that comes from being prepared can greatly improve the quality of your sleep, leaving you ready to tackle the next day with renewed energy.

And just as you might kick off your day with a dose of gratitude, make it a habit to end it in the same spirit. Reflect on what made you thankful today, no matter how small or grand. This practice not only caps off your day on a positive note but also sets the stage for a peaceful night's sleep and a hopeful new day.

From the motivational charge of "Get Off Your Ass" to the tranquility of "Sleep Hygiene," every step you take moves you closer to a healthier, more vibrant life using the M3 Method.

Picture this: Your day begins with a burst of energy and ends with serene rest, each moment curated to enhance every element of your life. With each idea and activity, you've built a day that not only celebrates movement but also honors rest, beautifully balancing action with rejuvenation.

We've just touched the surface of the importance of movement. The M3 Method will help you take this to a deeper and personal level with customized strategies tailored to your unique lifestyle and goals. This isn't just about following a set routine; it's about creating a personal journey that fits who you are and what you need, ensuring that every exercise, every mindful practice, and every moment of relaxation is tuned to your personal rhythm.

Embrace this holistic journey and let the M3 Method continue to guide you through each sunrise and sunset, crafting days as fulfilling as they are healthful. Dive deeper into the layers of movement and rest, exploring new dimensions of wellness that resonate with your individuality.

As you evolve within the M3 framework, you will discover the power of aligning daily actions with your personal aspirations, all designed to elevate your quality of life in profound ways.

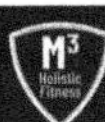

MOVEMENT ACTIONS

Review the following activities and complete at least three of them to help you integrate the Movement content into your life. Bonus points if you accomplish all of them.

1. Join a Movement Challenge: Commit to a 30-day movement challenge. Pick an activity that aligns with the MOVEMENT principles, track your progress, and share your experiences on social media using a specific hashtag to build a supportive community.

2. Mindful Momentum Journaling: Start a journal documenting how you incorporate mindful momentum into your daily activities. Reflect on how this changes your approach to physical fitness and overall well-being.

3. Explore and Share: Try a new form of movement this week (like yoga, Pilates, dancing, or hiking). Share your experience and insights in a blog post or social media to inspire others.

4. Body Awareness Meditation: Engage in a weekly body awareness meditation session. Focus on listening to your body's signals and write down your observations and feelings.

5. Weekly Diversified Workout Plan: Create a weekly workout plan that includes various types of exercises (cardio, strength, flexibility). Share your plan with a friend and encourage them to join you.

6. Experimentation Diary: Keep a diary of your exercise experiments. Note what works, what doesn't, and how each activity makes you feel, physically and emotionally.

7. Mind-Body Connection Class: Sign up for a class that focuses on connecting the mind and body, such as yoga or tai chi, and share your learnings with your community.

8. Natural Energy Boost Challenge: Replace one artificial stimulant (like caffeine) with a movement-based energy booster for a month and document the changes in your energy levels."

9. Movement as Self-Care Calendar:

- Create a monthly calendar where you schedule daily movement activities as a form of self-care. Share this calendar template with others.

- Consistency Tracker: Use an app or a physical tracker to monitor your movement consistency. Set goals, track your streaks, and reward yourself for milestones reached.

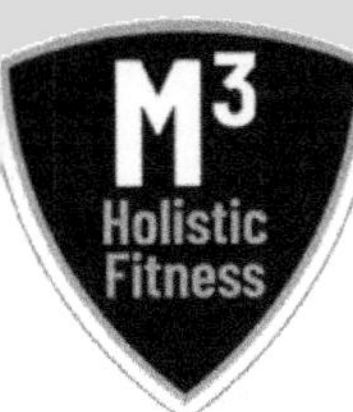

WHAT DOES YOUR LIFE LOOK LIKE?

1. Place a dot in each category to indicate your level of satisfaction within each area. A dot at the **center of the circle to indicate dissatisfaction**, or towards the **outer edge to indicate satisfaction**. Most people fall somewhere in between. (see example)

2. Connect the dots to see your **M₃ Circle of Life.**

3. Identify imbalances. Determine where to spend more time and energy to create balance. **This will help you create a better balance for your best Badass Life.**

SATISFACTION

DISSATISFACTION

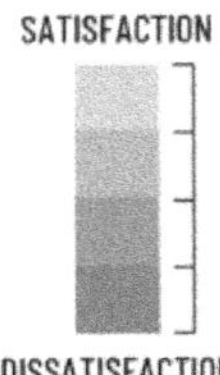

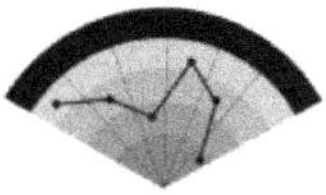

EXAMPLE

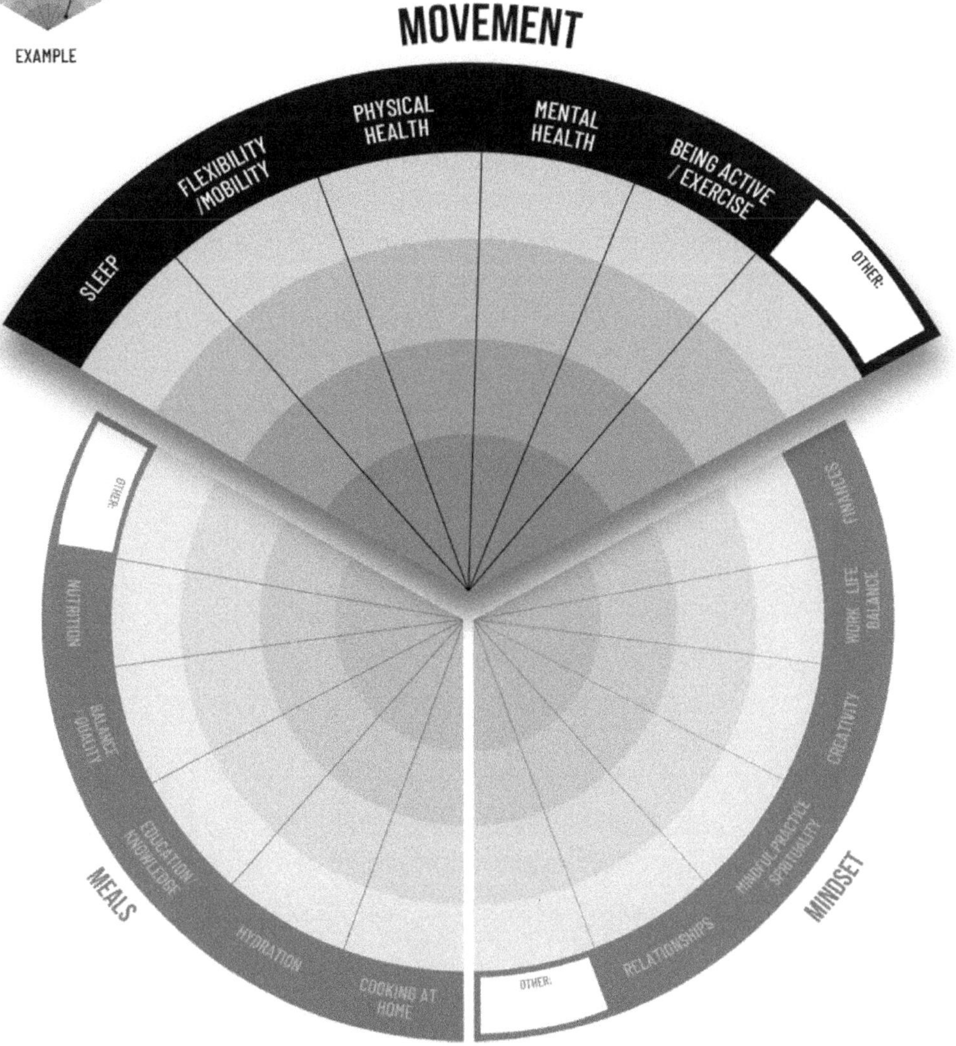

MOVEMENT

FREE DOWNLOAD

M3 Circle of Life Worksheet

http://dirkschultz.com/circle-of-life

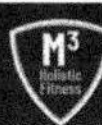

The M3 Method Shining Bright...

In the realm of fitness, there's a guiding light: The M3 Method, shining bright. It combines Mindset, Movement, and Meals, creating a holistic path for body and mind.

Set your thoughts with strength and grace, a resilient mindset, and your foundation in place. Embrace growth, let optimism flow, and see how you grow with every challenge.

Movement flows like a rhythmic song: Your body's dance, where you belong. From yoga's calm to cardio's fire, each step you take lifts you higher.

Meals that nourish, fuel your drive, with every bite, you feel alive. Whole foods, vibrant and fresh, Nourish your body, mind, and flesh.

Mindset strong, your thoughts align, Positive energy, a spark divine. Movement's joy, a lively beat, each motion made, a victory sweet.

Meals that heal, from farm to plate, nurture your soul, set you straight. Balanced choices, vibrant and true, Every dish, a gift to you.

The M3 Method, a life well-lived, with every day, more strength to give. Embrace this path, let it unfold, A journey to wellness, pure and bold.

So, rise each day with heart and cheer, The M3 Method always near. Mindset, Movement, Meals in blend, A radiant life, with joy no end.

THIS COULD BE...YOU!

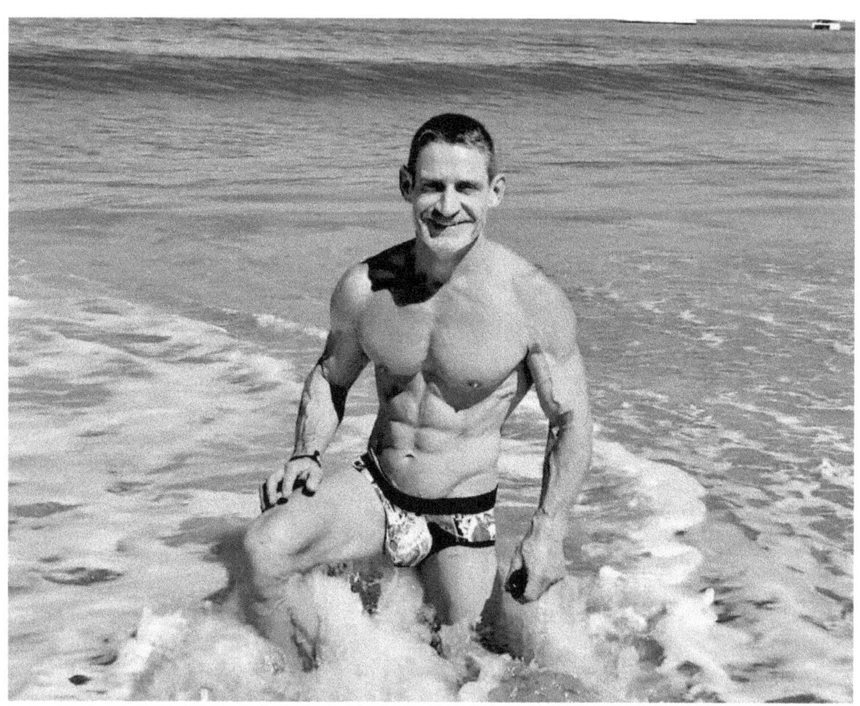

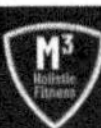

NOTES: WHAT DID YOU LEARN FROM THIS CHAPTER?

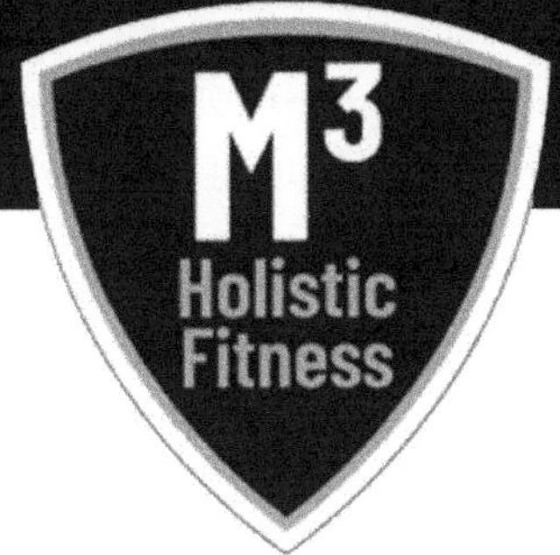

PART FOUR

MEALS

"If we could give every individual the right amount of nourishment and exercise, not too little and not too much, we would have found the safest way to health."
—Hippocrates circa 400 BC

M·E·A·L·S

Using the "MEALS" acronym, you can ensure a rounded, comprehensive view of nutrition in the context of holistic fitness and health.

M | Mindful Eating: Be present with every bite. Savoring flavors and textures help you appreciate your food, leading to healthier choices.

E | Energizing Nutrients: Choose foods that provide sustainable energy. Think whole grains, lean proteins, and beneficial fats to power both workouts and daily tasks. Think variety; eat from the rainbow.

A | Active Digestion: Prioritize foods that support digestive health. Incorporating probiotics, fiber-rich foods, and ample water can aid in the effective absorption of essential nutrients.

L | Lifestyle Balance: Balance your diet with other health pillars: consistent exercise, mental well-being, quality sleep, and emotional equilibrium.

S | Sustainable Choices: Opt for foods and eating practices that are sustainable both for your health, schedule, lifestyle, and the environment. This includes choosing local organic when possible and reducing waste to support a holistic approach to wellness.

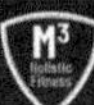

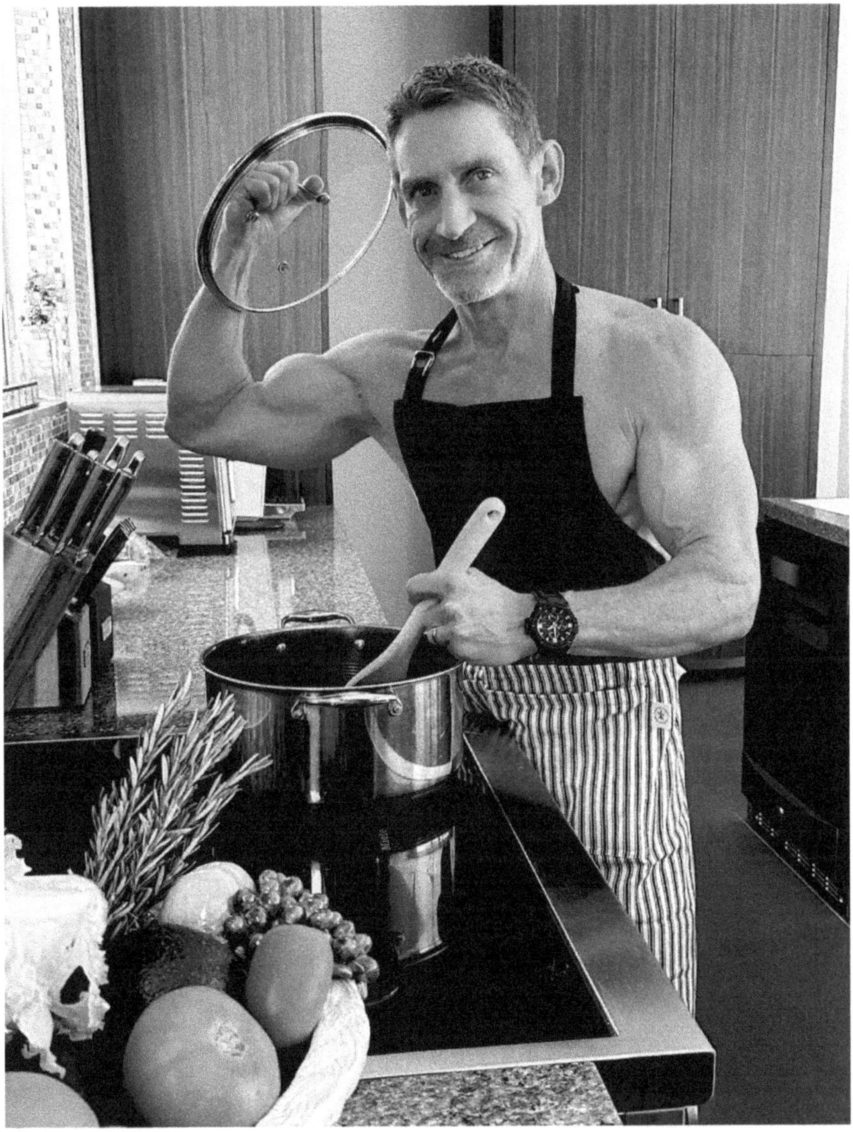

Meals

The Palette of Holistic Nourishment

"Let food be thy medicine and medicine be thy food."
—Hippocrates

Have you ever explored the depth of importance meals hold in our lives?

The food we eat goes beyond being just what we ingest to fuel our bodies. Nutritious, wholesome foods serve as the bedrock of our physical, mental, and emotional well-being, providing the essential energy and nutrients we need for peak performance. These foundational elements influence our physical health, rev up our energy levels, and even shape our mood and cognitive functions.

The food we eat not only nourishes our entire body but also supports the health of our gut microbiome: Think of your gut as the unsung hero in the story of your holistic well-being. It's not just a digestive chamber but a busy metropolis of trillions of bacteria cohabitating within you.

When this internal ecosystem thrives, it's like having a harmonious community inside of you. The residents—those countless bacteria—live in peaceful coexistence with your body, providing an array of perks. These advantages range from streamlining your digestive processes for more consistent bowel movements to fine-tuning your immune defenses. They even play a role in regulating your mood and appetite.

Just as nutritious meals and diverse forms of nourishment enrich your life, a balanced gut microbiome contributes its own set of benefits, adding another layer of depth and complexity to your holistic health journey. It's another essential element that holds greater importance as we age.

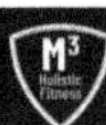

But there's more to the story. Beyond the sustenance that food provides, there are other forms of nourishment that add depth, texture, and richness to our lives. Think of nurturing relationships that satisfy our craving for connection, meaningful work that stokes our sense of purpose, and creative outlets that spark our imagination. Let's not forget spiritual practices that quench our thirst for inner peace and a sense of meaning.

Each of these elements offers its own unique form of nourishment, enriching not just our bodies but also our minds, hearts, and souls. They elevate our day-to-day experiences, bringing joy and fulfillment, and contribute to an overarching sense of well-being.

In shaping the artistry of our lives, the concept of Meals extends to everything that nourishes us, both literally and metaphorically. As we layer our days with these various forms of nourishment, we craft a well-rounded, balanced, and holistic portrait of health. Just as an artist skillfully blends different elements to realize their vision, integrating these nourishments enables us to sculpt our holistic well-being, allowing us to live our lives to the fullest.

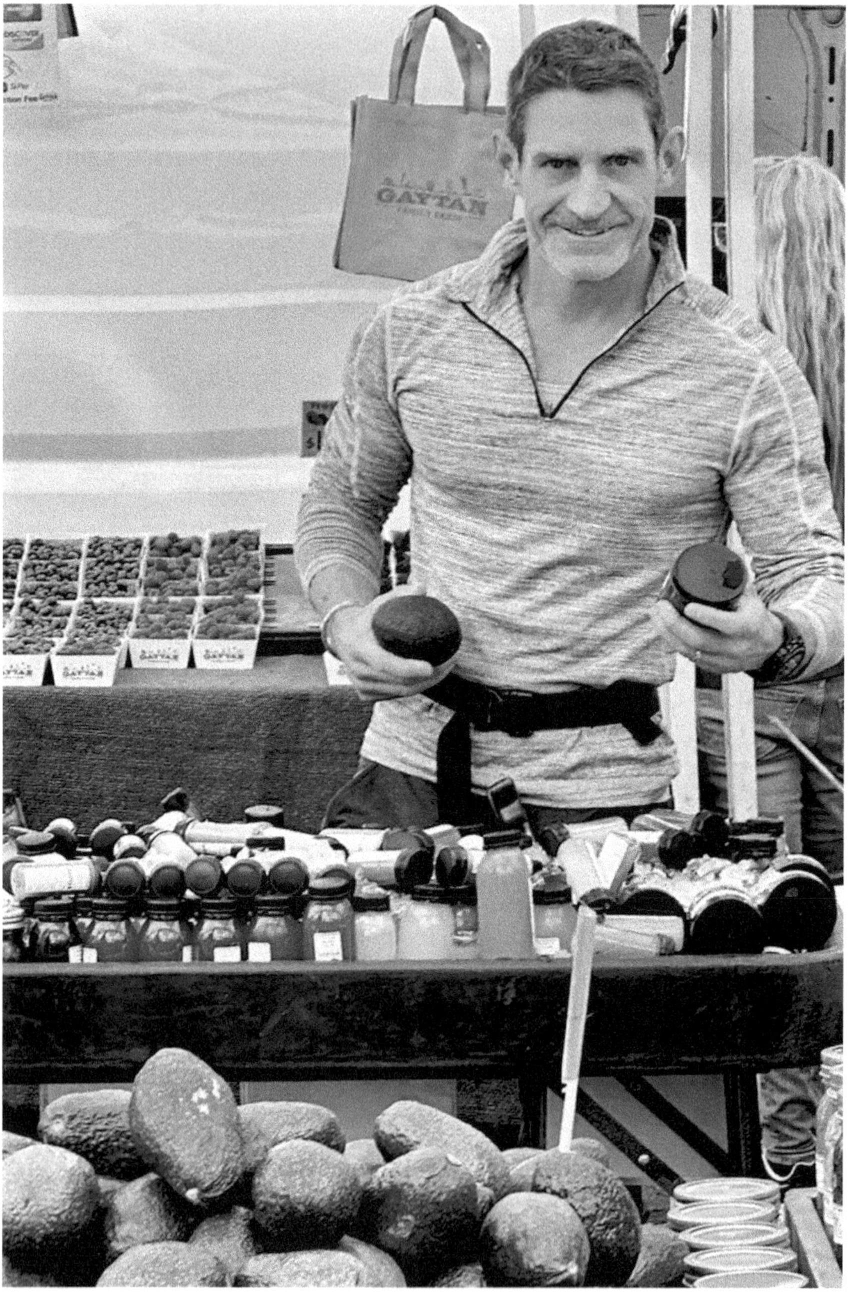

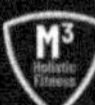

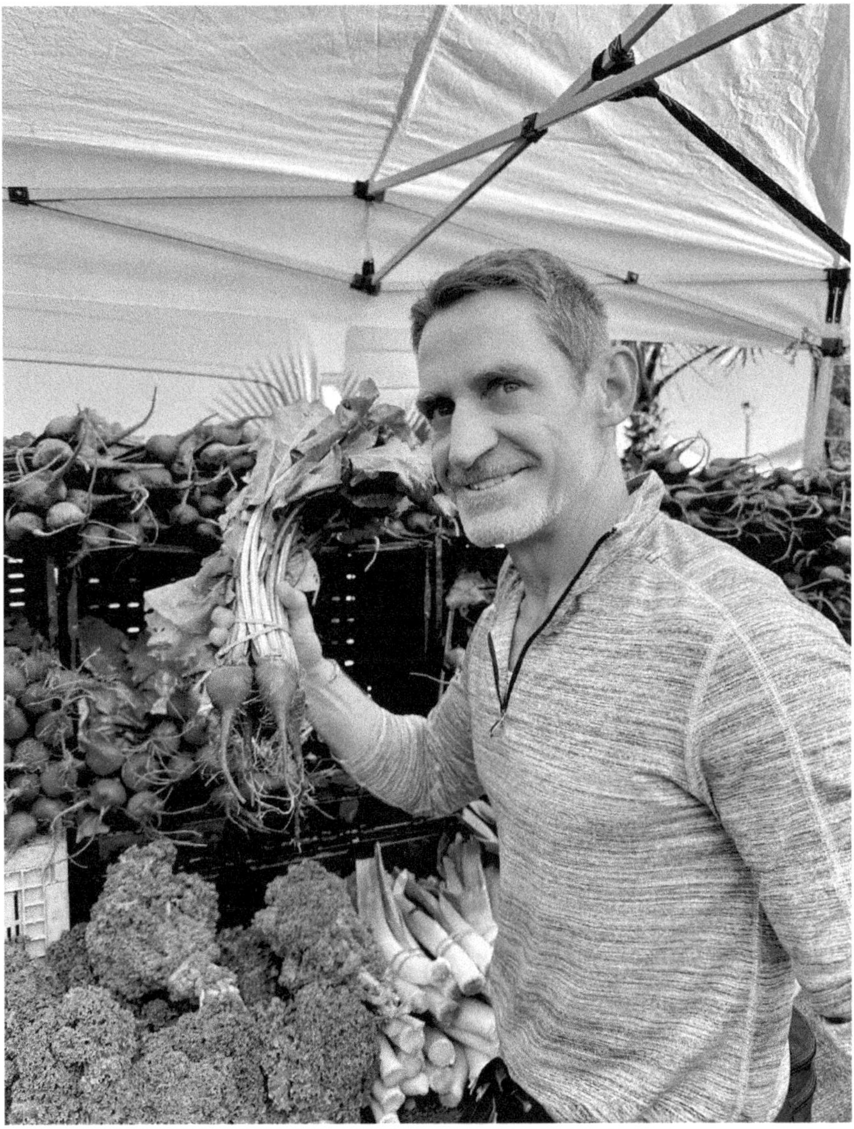

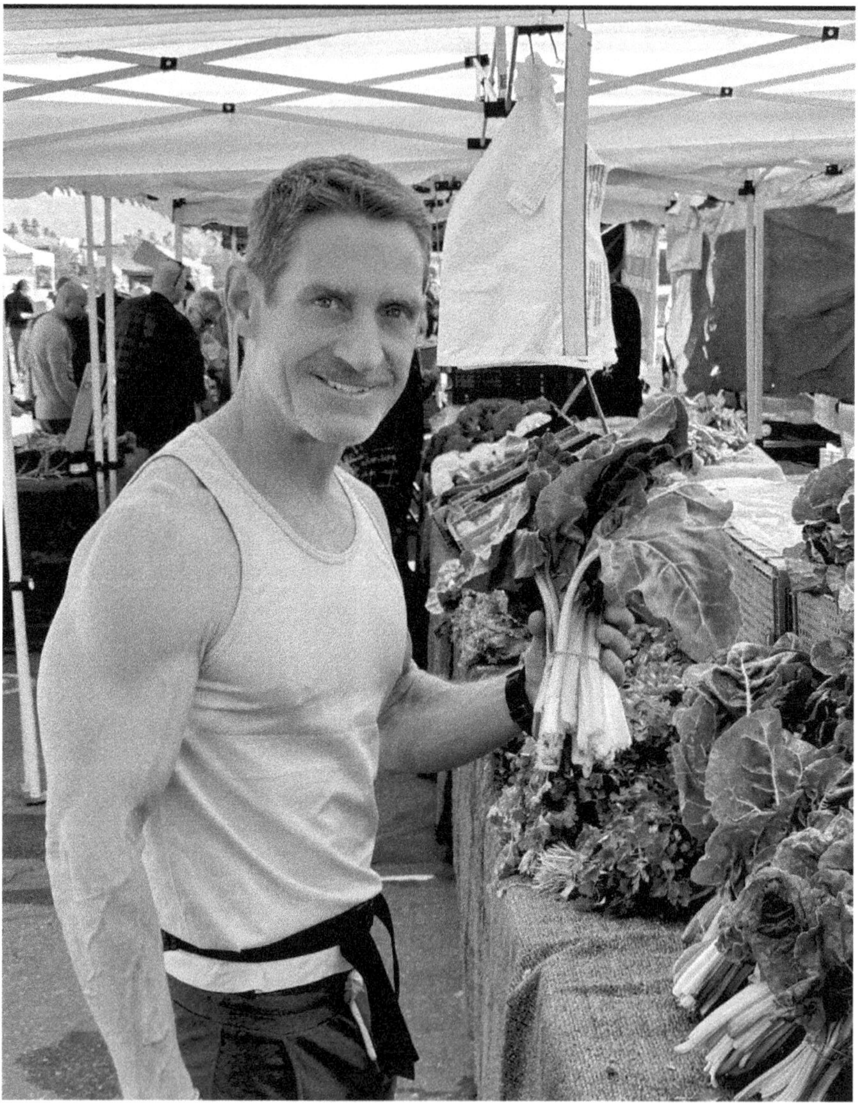

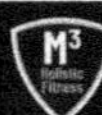

THE 5 ELEMENTS OF MEALS

It's time to explore the five elements of meals that make every dish a masterpiece of health and flavor! These aren't just ingredients; they're the cornerstones of the M3 Mindset eating philosophy.

- Cooking at Home

- Hydration

- Education

- Balance & Quality

- Nutrition

Together, these elements transform eating from a mundane task into an exhilarating journey towards wellness. Let's explore how each one plays a role in crafting a life rich in taste and health!

1 — COOKING AT HOME

Meals are more than just fuel; they're a heartfelt connection to your wellness journey.

Home cooking isn't just about making food; it's about whipping up some magic in your own kitchen—fun, flirty, and absolutely sexy. Who doesn't love someone who can cook? When you cook at home, you're not just tossing ingredients together; you're actively shaping your health and creating heartfelt connections to your wellness journey.

Every step in the kitchen, from selecting organic veggies to balancing macronutrients, puts you firmly in charge of your dietary path. You get to choose every ingredient with care, ensuring each one aligns with your health standards and goals. By steering clear of processed foods and exploring various cooking methods like steaming, roasting, and even fermenting, you elevate the health benefits of your meals.

Adding herbs and spices not only cranks up the flavor but also amps up the antioxidant power of your dishes, turning each meal into a vibrant feast for your senses. Cooking at home is your health strategy disguised as culinary fun, where every dish you prepare is an opportunity to cut out processed sugars, unhealthy fats, and artificial additives.

Think of your kitchen as your personal wellness retreat, where every meal crafted is a step towards a more vibrant, health-conscious life. So, tie on that apron—it's time to make some magic happen, one delicious meal at a time!

Mindful Nutrition

Think of mindful nutrition as your secret ingredient in the kitchen. It's not just about filling your plate; it's about fueling your entire well-being. Your kitchen? That's your playground. Here, you're free to mix things up, get creative, and really dive into what makes food good for both body and soul.

Choosing organic produce isn't just about being trendy—it's about being smart. You dodge those sneaky pesticides and synthetic nasties, ensuring every ingredient is as fresh and natural as possible. This way, you're not just eating—you're fortifying your body with all the essential nutrients it craves.

And hey, your kitchen is more than a place to whip up meals; it's where you become a culinary wizard. Experiment with flavors, play with spices, and transform simple ingredients into magic on a plate. This is where you turn your health goals into delicious realities, one tasty dish at a time. So, grab those herbs, fire up the stove, and let's make eating well the highlight of your day!

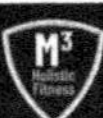

Meat Matters

Quality is king when it comes to meat. Grass-fed, grass-finished beef, for example, is a nutritional powerhouse. This type of beef is significantly richer in omega-3 fatty acids, which are essential for heart health and reducing inflammation. Omega-3s can also support brain function and improve mood. Additionally, grass-fed beef contains higher levels of vitamin E, a powerful antioxidant that protects your cells from damage and supports a healthy immune system. Another key component is conjugated linoleic acid (CLA), which has been shown to help with fat loss, muscle retention, and even cancer prevention.

Pasture-raised eggs and chicken offer their own set of unique nutritional benefits. Eggs from pasture-raised hens typically contain higher levels of omega-3 fatty acids, vitamin A, vitamin E, and beta-carotene compared to their conventionally raised counterparts. These nutrients contribute to eye health, skin health, and overall immune function.

Similarly, pasture-raised chicken is leaner and has a better fat profile, including more omega-3s and less saturated fat. The humane and natural raising practices also result in meat that's free from antibiotics and hormones, providing a cleaner and more nutritious option for your meals.

By choosing high-quality, pasture-raised meats and eggs, you not only enhance the nutritional value of your meals but also support sustainable farming practices that are better for the environment and animal welfare. This holistic approach to meat consumption ensures you're fueling your body with the best possible nutrients while making a positive impact on the world around you.

Plant-Based

For all the vegetarians and vegans out there, your kitchen is more than just a place to cook—it's your very own culinary stage where you get to express your creativity with food. It's where you get to whip up nutrient-packed, flavorful meals that align with your values. Dive into the art of plant-based cooking and make sure you're stacking your dishes with plenty of protein, iron, calcium, and all those vital nutrients your body craves.

And don't just wing it! There's a whole world of resources at your fingertips. Crack open some books, scroll through websites, and check out the flood of plant-based blogs bursting with recipes, meal plans, and nutritional advice tailored just for you. These resources are gold mines for learning how to balance your diet and keep your body humming happily on a vegan or vegetarian lifestyle. So, start exploring and turn your meal prep into an adventure in healthy eating!

Sugar Is Not Your Friend

Heads up, sweet tooth gang! While those scrumptious cookies and decadent cakes might seem like a treat, they're actually tough on your health. Refined sugar, the not-so-sweet villain behind these goodies, isn't just an indulgence—it's a major health trap, especially as you step into the golden years.

And let's not overlook carbs like bread and pasta, which sneakily transform into sugar in your body, mimicking the effects of the sweet stuff. They spike your blood sugar, bringing on the dreaded crash and craving cycle. So maybe think twice before reaching for that extra slice of pizza or that second helping of spaghetti.

Sugar is sneaky—it not only messes with your energy levels but can also pack on pounds and pave the way for type

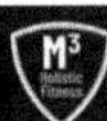

2 diabetes and heart disease. Plus, it's a pro at speeding up the aging process, affecting everything from the plumpness of your skin to your overall vascular health. Next time you're tempted by that frosted cupcake or sugar-laden latte, remember what's at stake. It could make it a whole lot easier to choose the apple over the apple pie.

Sugar also loves to play hide and seek on food labels, disguising itself with all sorts of names. Watch out for sneaky terms like corn syrup, dextrose, fructose, and many others that are essentially sugar in disguise. Educating yourself about these aliases can help you dodge the hidden sugar bullet in your diet.

So, what can you do to cut down? Start simple: skip dessert, opt for less candy, and reach for fruits when you need a sweet fix. Remember to scrutinize labels to sidestep those hidden sugars. It might be a bit of a challenge at first—sugar is addictive, after all!

But stick with it, and you'll notice you're feeling more vibrant and balanced. Your mood will lift, and your body will definitely be happier. So, forego the soda, say no to that candy bar, and become a label-reading pro. Trust me, your body will thank you!

The Road to Easier Cooking

If the thought of cooking makes you sweat more than a spicy jalapeño, don't worry—meal prep kits and services are here to save the day! Take some time to scout out which ones match your palate and health goals. Embrace the savvy "cook once, eat twice" strategy to maximize your kitchen efforts, turning one cooking session into several scrumptious meals.

If you want to make meal prep a whole lot easier, how about hosting themed dinner parties? Pick a cuisine for each gathering—Italian, Thai, Mexican, you name it. Your friends choose the dish and do the cooking, and you set the food quality standards, keeping it fun and healthy. It's a fun and delicious way to spice up your meal prep and enjoy great food with friends, and you get to keep the leftovers.

Think of each ingredient and choice you make in the kitchen as a brushstroke on your personal health masterpiece. Nutrition isn't one-size-fits-all; it's as unique as your fingerprint. Explore and experiment to find what fuels your body best and paint your own vibrant picture of health and happiness.

2 — HYDRATION

Hydration is one of the easiest yet most overlooked aspects of health. Staying properly hydrated is the bedrock of your body's intricate systems, and it's incredibly simple to improve.

Water is the elixir of life, and for good reason. It does more than just quench your thirst—it hydrates every cell, organ, and system in your body, acting as the silent hero behind all your physiological processes. Your body is mostly water, and this fluid medium is essential for countless biochemical reactions. From energy production and nutrient distribution to waste elimination, hydration is the unsung facilitator of your overall health. Keeping yourself well-hydrated fuels your metabolism, sharpens your mind, and optimizes nutrient delivery.

When it comes to water, quality matters. Just as you choose whole, organic foods, you should ensure your water is clean and free from contaminants like heavy metals, chlorine, and pollutants. This way, you're replenishing your body without introducing harmful agents.

Think of hydration as your body's natural detox champion. Your kidneys rely on adequate hydration to flush out toxins efficiently. And the benefits extend beyond internal cleans-

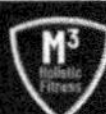

ing—proper hydration gives you radiant skin, smooth digestion, and even a mood boost. On the flip side, even mild dehydration can trigger headaches, fatigue, and mental fog.

Everyone's hydration needs vary based on factors like climate, activity level, age, and individual health conditions. But a general rule of thumb is around 90-126 ounces daily. In the M3 Method, hydration is a fundamental pillar of your wellness journey.

Proper hydration keeps your red blood cells agile, allowing them to maneuver through the tiniest capillaries and efficiently distribute oxygen. Without enough fluids, these cells become sluggish, compromising your energy levels and cellular health.

Think of hydration as an intentional act of self-care. Each gulp is more than a reflex—it's a conscious affirmation of your commitment to nourishing yourself deeply and fundamentally.

Not all beverages are created equal when it comes to hydration. Coffee, teas, sodas, and juices have varied impacts on your hydration status. While coffee and caffeinated teas can act as diuretics, sugary sodas, and juices add empty calories and can promote dehydration.

Your morning coffee might wake you up, but too much can lead to dehydration. It's not just about the caffeine; excess sugar in sodas and juices can compound dehydration and derail your health goals.

It's important to become aware of the effects of what you drink and remember that pure water should always be your go-to. Water remains the unmatched champion in hydrating and supporting your body's myriad functions. Make it the cornerstone of your hydration strategy while treating other beverages as occasional guest stars, consumed mindfully and in moderation.

3 — EDUCATION

Diving into the ever-evolving world of nutrition and wellness is like enrolling in a lifelong course where every day brings new lessons and discoveries. As science unfolds and cultures shift, keeping your knowledge fresh and updated is not just helpful—it's crucial. Think of nutrition as a lively debate club where yesterday's health villains, like dietary fats, get a chance to clean up their reputations and prove their worth with solid, research-backed benefits.

It's a big, tasty world out there! From the heart-friendly fares of the Mediterranean diet to the time-tested wisdom of Ayurvedic meals, being well-informed lets you cherry-pick the best from global eating habits to spice up your own meal plans. This isn't just about eating differently; it's about enriching your dietary canvas with colors and flavors that enhance your health and zest for life.

The intersection between meals and lifestyle choices is hard to overlook. The when, where, and how of your meals can transform your dining table into a cornerstone of wellness. Keeping up with the latest research about when to eat and how to prepare your plate not only helps you make smarter choices but also integrates these insights into a lifestyle that's as wholesome as it is enjoyable.

In this information age, your greatest tool is discernment—filtering the fads from the facts can feel like hunting for treasures in the digital wild. The M3 Method isn't just your guide; it's your compass in navigating the maze of superfoods and diet trends, helping you to distill pure, actionable knowledge.

Education in nutrition and wellness is more than accumulating facts; it's an active, vibrant pursuit of knowledge. It challenges you to adapt, personalize, and refine your approach as you grow. Remember, what works for one may not work for another.

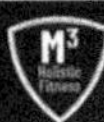

"One person's food is another's poison."

Embrace this journey of continuous learning, and let it sculpt a healthier, more enlightened you. Every bite, every meal becomes a step towards mastering the art of living well.

4 — BALANCE AND QUALITY

Diving into good nutrition isn't just about watching calories or sticking to a diet plan—it's about mastering the perfect blend of discipline and pleasure in your eating habits.

Think of your meal plan as your nutritional anchor; it's your rock-solid foundation that consistently fuels your body with essential nutrients to keep you at the top of your game. And when it comes to ingredients, quality is key. Choosing organic, fresh, and sustainably sourced isn't just trendy—it's a health-smart decision that maximizes the benefits of every bite you take.

But life's too delicious to stick only to the script on your meal prep chart. The world's culinary stage is vast and varied, from the spicy thrill of a Thai curry to the comforting embrace of an Italian risotto, or the rich, intricate layers of a Moroccan tagine. Each dish isn't just a treat for your taste buds; it's an expansion of your nutritional repertoire.

Now, here's the real spice: tuning into your body's own signals. It's like having an internal compass that points you to what your body loves and what it doesn't, helping you dodge the foods that drag you down and embrace those that make you feel fantastic. Listening to your body helps you tailor your meals to be as nourishing as they are enjoyable.

Balance and quality in your diet create a symphony of great health. By anchoring yourself in a consistent, quality-filled meal plan while leaving room for culinary adventures, you're playing a smarter, more soul-satisfying game of nutrition. This approach doesn't just fuel your body; it feeds your spirit, reminding you that eating well is about delighting in the science and the spontaneity of food.

5 — NUTRITION

When it comes to nutrition, think of it as both the cornerstone of aging gracefully and the ultimate game-changer for your health. Sure, food is your body's fuel, but let's elevate the conversation: it's also your preventative powerhouse, your healing agent, and your ticket to thriving in the long game of life.

Nutritional mindfulness isn't just about savoring the flavors; it's about developing a discerning palate that knows the difference between what nourishes you and what weakens you. Think vibrant veggies, sun-kissed fruits, lean proteins, and foods as close to nature as possible. Whole, unprocessed foods enhance your body's natural systems, from giving your immune response a power-up and sharpening your cognitive edge to making every cell in your body feel like it just hit the jackpot.

Highly processed foods rob you of your nutrition, and sodas are not just empty calories; they're calcium thieves that weaken your bones over time. And let's not forget how sneaky sugar can be, hiding in processed goodies and messing with nutrient absorption, laying down the red carpet for health issues. Pass on desserts, eat less candy, and read labels to make healthier choices. And remember, bread, pasta, and other carbs that convert to sugar have the same effect as refined sugar.

Another offender on the list? Trans fats are the bad boys of the dietary world. Notorious for their heart-harming effects, they also mess with your omega-3 absorption, which is like throwing a wrench into your brain health and anti-inflammatory functions. Speaking of life's indulgences, too much

alcohol doesn't just throw shade at your liver; it can drain your B vitamins and essential minerals, setting the stage for cognitive fog, chronic tiredness, and a not-so-stellar immune system.

Knowledge is your superpower. Once you're aware of nutritionally empty foods, you can actively sidestep them. This wisdom isn't just a nice-to-have; it's non-negotiable. It's your roadmap to a life bursting with vitality, strength, and holistic awesomeness.

The most important nutrient is oxygen because it is essential for every cell in your body to function properly. Oxygen fuels your cells, supports cellular respiration, and helps in energy production. This is why exercise is so vital; it increases your heart rate and breathing, delivering more oxygen to your entire body. Regular physical activity ensures that your muscles, organs, and tissues receive the oxygen they need to operate at their best, promoting overall health and well-being.

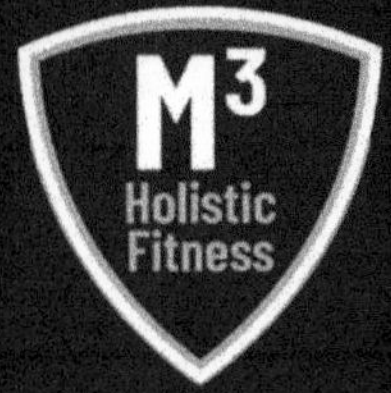

ON THE PLATE · OFF THE PLATE

You've probably heard the phrase "you are what you eat," and it holds a kernel of truth that goes beyond the plate. Nutrition isn't just the fuel that powers your biological engines; it's a holistic practice that nourishes your body and soul. The M3 Method elevates this concept, embracing a comprehensive approach to nutrition that focuses not only on the food on your plate but also on the nourishment off the plate— the many forms that feed your spirit, mind, and emotional well-being.

On your plate, the focus is on choosing foods that boost your health and vitality. This means balancing macronutrients—proteins, fats, and carbohydrates—with a rich array of vitamins and minerals from fruits, vegetables, whole grains, and lean proteins. Making informed food choices enhances your physical functions and supports your long-term health.

Off the plate, the concept of meals includes the intellectual, emotional, and spiritual sustenance you gather from your daily experiences. This might be the joy found in meaningful relationships, the intellectual spark from engaging in hobbies, or the tranquility discovered in spiritual practices like meditation. In the M3 Method, these elements are as crucial to your health as the food you consume.

By expanding the definition of meals to encompass all the ways you nourish yourself, the M3 Method promotes a holistic view of health. It acknowledges the importance of feeding your mind and spirit alongside your body, fostering a balanced, vibrant, and fulfilling life. This comprehensive approach to well-being ensures that every aspect of your life is nurtured, leading to a more harmonious and healthful existence.

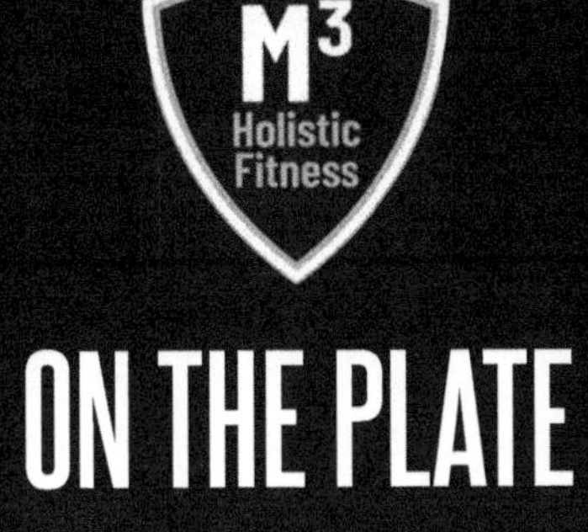

ON THE PLATE

Nutritional Balance for Optimal Health

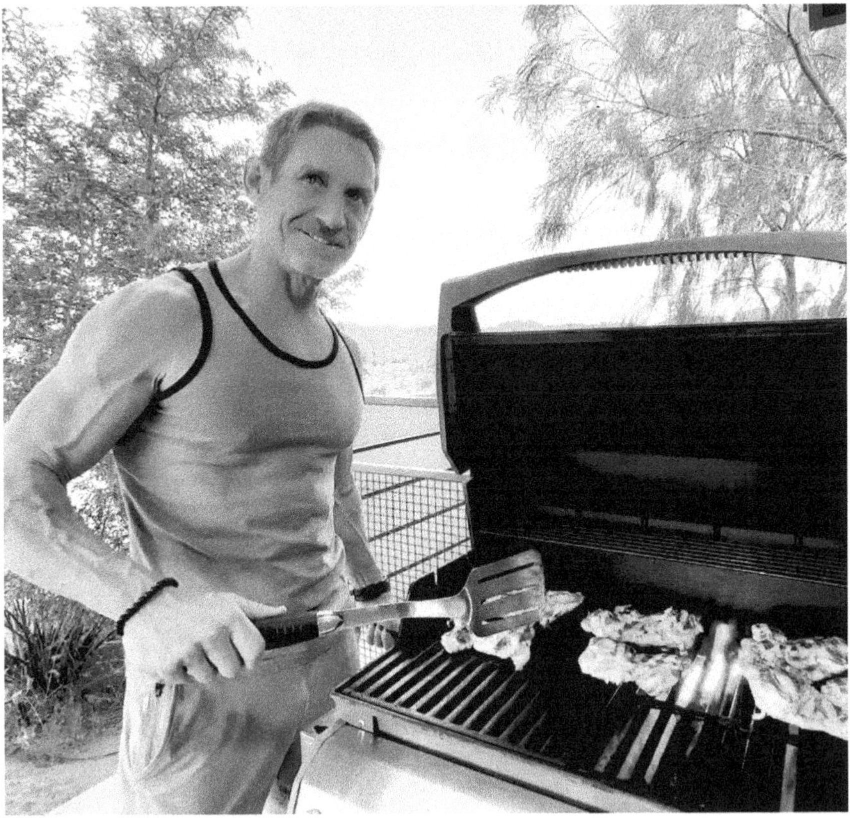

F.O.O.D.

The food you put on your plate nourishes not just your body but also impacts your mental health and energy levels. Understanding this connection empowers you to make choices that enhance your every aspect of your overall health and well-being.

A balanced diet plays a critical role in your health—it can reduce the risk of chronic diseases, bolster digestion, support your immune system, elevate your mood, and significantly improve your quality of life.

To help you remember the essential principles of nourishing both your body and mind with your dietary choices, let's dive into the acronym for "FOOD." This will guide you through focusing on what truly matters when it comes to eating right and living well.

F — Focus on quality fuel

O — Out with the "bullshit" food

O — Observe what your body needs

D — Decide to eat with intention: Mindful Eating

F | Focus on quality fuel: Make whole, anti-inflammatory, and energy-rich foods the foundation of your diet. Opt for fresh, unprocessed ingredients that provide essential nutrients and support recovery and optimal performance. Foods low on the glycemic index offer more sustained energy and promote long—term health.

O | Out with the "bullshit" food: Eliminate or limit processed foods and seed oils and the "three white devils": processed sugar, salt, and white flour. These ingredients can contribute to inflammation, weight gain, and various health issues. Prioritize nutrient-dense, whole foods to support your overall well-being.

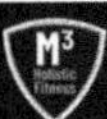

O | Observe what your body needs: Recognize that your nutritional needs may change at different stages of your life. Embrace the concept of bio-individuality, understanding that what works for one person may not work for another. Pay attention to how your body reacts to different foods and adjust your diet accordingly to optimize your health.

D | Decide to eat with intention: Mindful Eating: Incorporating mindful eating into your daily routine involves more than just choosing nutritious foods; it's also about how you eat. Start by eating with intention, selecting foods that will nourish both your body and mind. As you eat, take the time to slow down and truly savor each bite, making a conscious effort to put down your fork between mouthfuls. Engage all of your senses as you eat, appreciating the colors, textures, smells, and flavors that make up your meal. It's also crucial to check in with yourself during your meal, asking questions like, "How hungry am I?" to gauge your appetite and prevent overeating.

Let's be practical about how you approach your meals.

First, cut down on distractions during mealtime—turn off the TV, put your phone away, and focus on your food. This not only helps you enjoy your meal more but also makes you more aware of what and how much you're eating. Keep a positive attitude about food; it can make a huge difference in your eating habits. Negative thinking can derail your progress, so focus on the good stuff.

When it comes to portion sizes, try the 80% rule. Stop eating when you feel about 80% full. It takes about 20-30 minutes for your brain to catch up with your stomach, so give it time to signal that you're full.

Watch your alcohol intake—enjoy it in moderation and be mindful of its impact on your health. And while you're at it, keep an eye on caffeine and added sugars. Too much can mess with your energy levels and lead to weight gain.

By following these tips, summed up in the "FOOD" acronym, you'll make smarter dietary choices and develop a healthier relationship with food. Remember, it's all about finding the right balance between nourishment and enjoyment, making your meals a mindful and fulfilling part of your day.

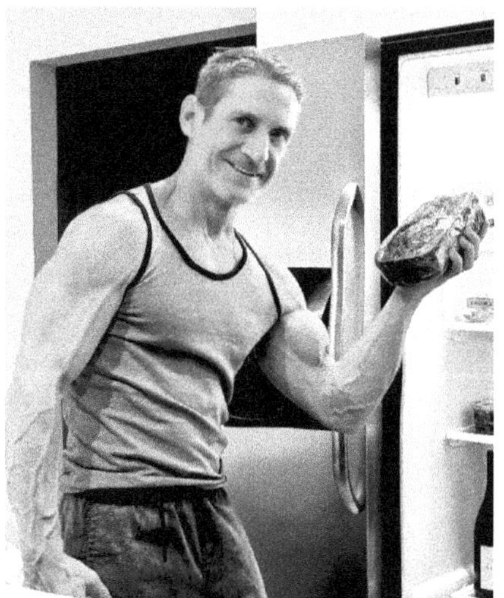
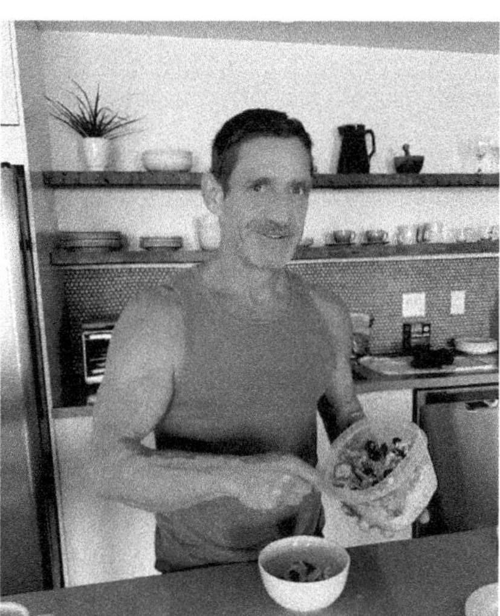

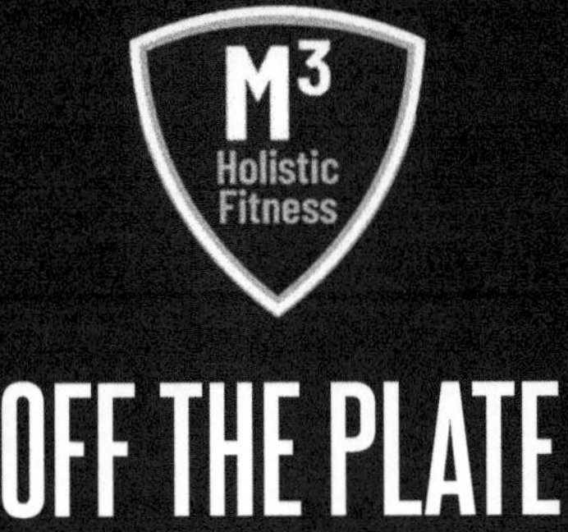

OFF THE PLATE

Environment & Relationships

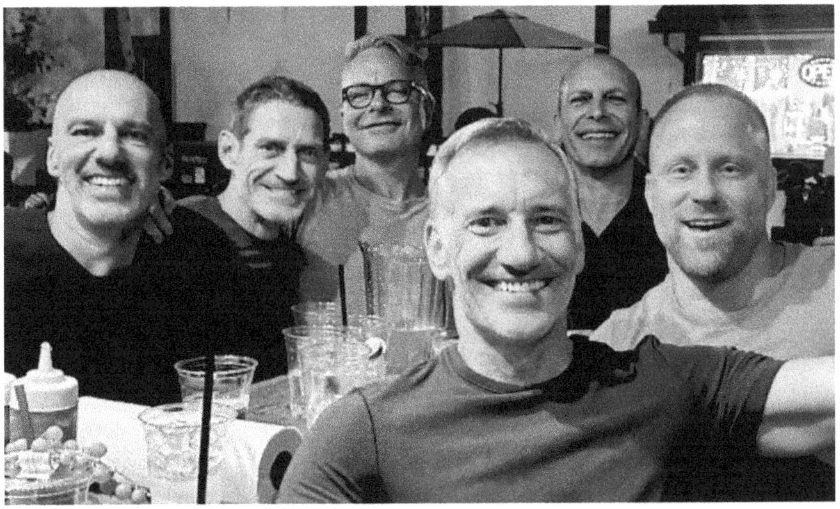

Overall Environment

Let's talk about "Meals off the Plate" and how our emotional environment is just as crucial as the food we eat.

Our well-being isn't just about what we eat but also about the people we surround ourselves with. Think about your friends and acquaintances. Do they bring positivity and lift you up? Being around people who make you feel good is like filling your plate with nutritious, vibrant foods. These relationships, built on genuine understanding and shared goals, are like lifelines. Their support, kindness, and laughter nourish us, acting as essential vitamins and minerals for our mental and emotional health.

Our work environment matters too. A positive work setting is like the main course of a balanced meal. It's all about mutual respect, constructive feedback, and teamwork. This kind of environment fuels our ambition and strengthens our sense of self-worth. In these spaces, we feel valued and inspired to reach our potential.

In today's digital world, the media we consume is like a big buffet of visuals, stories, and information. There's a ton of TV shows, movies, and online content out there, ranging from inspiring to negative. Just like a buffet offers both nourishing dishes and less healthy options, too much focus on negativity or violence in what we watch and read can be like junk food for the soul, sapping our emotional well-being.

It's important to be selective about what we consume with our minds, choosing only content that uplifts and educates, filling our minds with positivity, knowledge, and inspiration.

The places we live, the books we read, the hobbies we pursue, and our daily rituals all shape our well-being. They're like the side dishes that add flavor to our lives. Be as selective about your surroundings and activities as you are about your diet, choosing those that bring joy and growth.

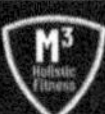

While the foods we eat sustain our bodies, the emotional environments and content we choose nurture our souls. Recognizing and curating these "Meals off the Plate" leads to a life well-lived.

Relationship Environment

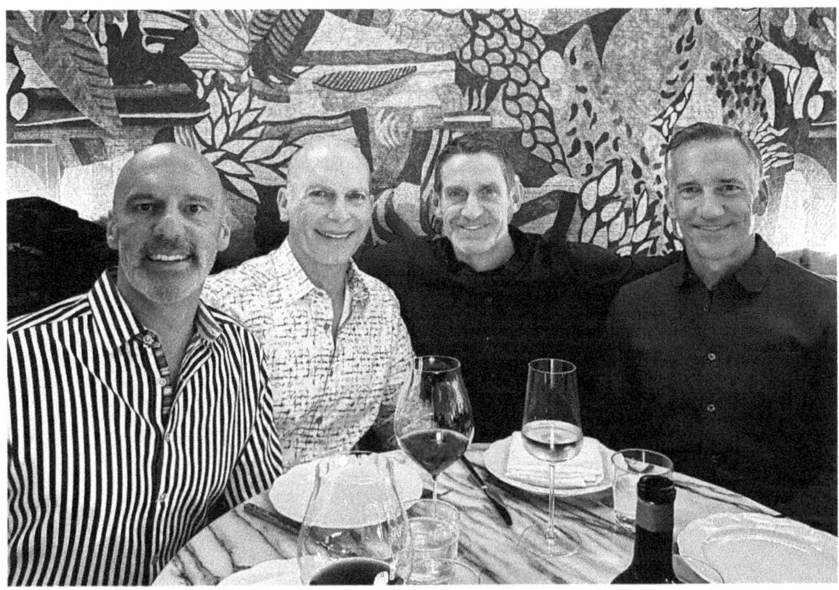

Just as a good meal fills you up and keeps you going, healthy relationships provide the love, support, and sense of belonging that help you flourish. When relationships are rocky, they can really drag you down. But when they're healthy? They're like soul food—packed with love, empathy, and deep connections that really lift your spirits and remind you that you're never alone when you've got great people in your corner.

At the core of every solid relationship are shared interests and values, mutual respect, trust, and open communication. Whether it's with your significant other, a dear friend, or family members, these connections become your personal sanctuaries. In these relationships, you get to grow together, share your deepest fears without judgment, and face life's challenges together. You'll celebrate successes, cheer on dreams, and build a support network that's rock solid. Cherish these bonds, nurture them, and let them boost your life, knowing there's always someone rooting for you.

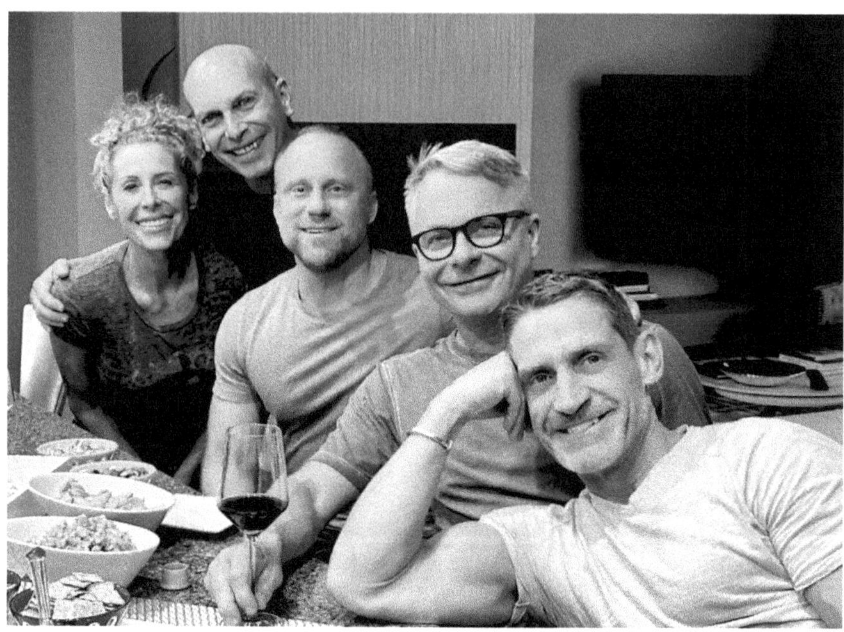

Just like junk food can wreck your health, unhealthy relationships can cast long shadows over your life. Filled with mistrust, disrespect, or manipulation, these toxic ties are like empty calories—temporarily filling but ultimately unfulfilling. They can leave you feeling drained, unhappy, or inadequate. Whether it's controlling romantic relationships, one-sided friendships, or tense family dynamics, these relationships can stir up stress, anxiety, and plenty of negativity.

Spotting these harmful dynamics is the first step to protecting your emotional health. Sometimes, moving forward might mean seeking professional help to work through complex issues. Other times, it might mean making the tough decision to cut ties for the sake of your peace of mind. And sometimes, with enough effort and mutual willingness, even strained relationships can be healed.

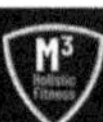

Relationships are a huge part of life's rich tapestry. They can either nourish your soul or deplete your energy, so making thoughtful choices about who you let into your life is key. By fostering and valuing healthy connections, you keep your emotional and mental health vibrant, allowing you to enjoy a life filled with joy, purpose, and deep satisfaction. Always prioritize relationships that lift you up, and don't shy away from reevaluating the ones that don't. Your emotional well-being is absolutely worth it.

Home Environment

Your home environment plays an enormous role in your well-being—it's not just about keeping it clean; it's about creating a space that supports your mental and emotional health. Think of your living space as a reflection of your inner state; when it's organized, you feel organized, too.

Imagine stepping into your home and feeling an instant wave of calm wash over you. That's the magic of a clean, peaceful living space. It's a comfy retreat from the hustle of life where you can truly unwind. Picture a tidy living room with cozy furniture, soft lighting, and a couple of houseplants that bring a bit of nature indoors. This kind of setup doesn't just look inviting—it genuinely boosts your mood and provides a sanctuary where you can relax, recharge, and gear up for whatever comes next.

So, how can you make this vision a reality? It's more than just about good looks. A well-kept, serene home not only looks great but also lifts your spirits. Start with something small—clear off those kitchen counters or set up a snug reading nook by the window. Imagine sinking into a comfy chair, with a good book and a cup of tea, bathed in gentle sunlight. It's these small touches that can minimize stress and make your home truly welcoming.

Take a moment to look around your living space. Does it feel like a haven of peace and happiness? If not, it might be time for a little tweaking. Bring in some greenery with a few houseplants, tackle that cluttered spare room, or throw open the windows to flood your home with fresh air and sunlight. These simple changes can make a big difference, turning your house into a real sanctuary. After all, it's all about creating a home that looks good, feels good, and perfectly suits your lifestyle.

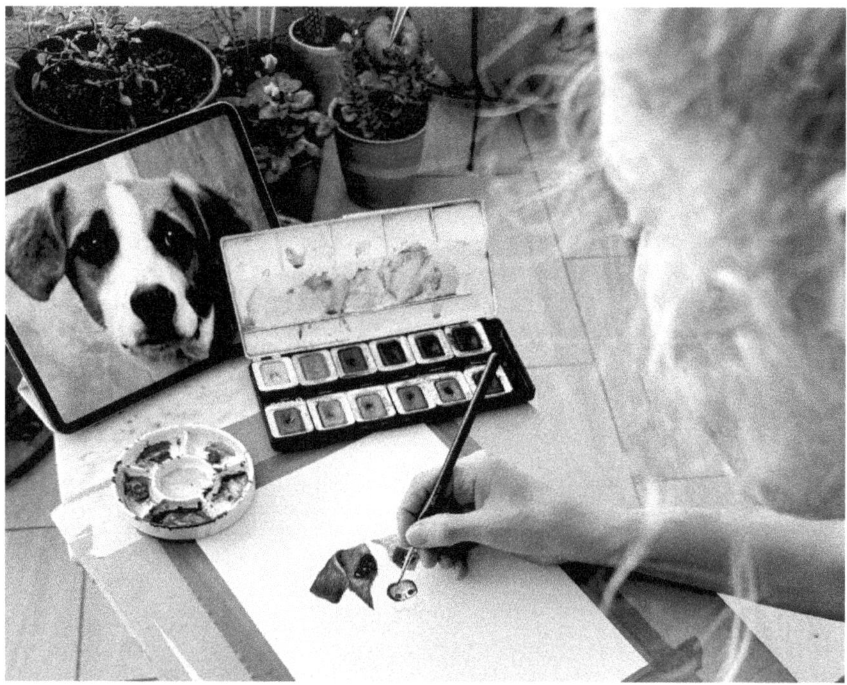

On the flip side, a cluttered and chaotic home can really crank up your stress levels. We've all been there—feeling swamped by mess and noise. It's more than just uncomfortable; it's actually bad for your health. So why not make it a priority to create a more harmonious home? Start by decluttering to bring some order, add some plants for a touch of tranquility, and carve out cozy nooks where you can kick back and relax. Picture transforming your bedroom into a peaceful sanctuary where you can truly unwind after a hectic day.

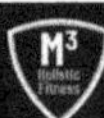

Really, the state of your home can either lift you up or drag you down. By paying attention to its impact and making thoughtful tweaks, you can craft a space that boosts your well-being. Take a good look around—does your space inspire you to be your best? If not, it's time to make those small yet powerful changes. Maybe it's rearranging the furniture to create a better flow, adding a few cheerful decor items, or turning your bedroom into a quiet escape. These adjustments can make a huge difference, helping you forge a nurturing environment that supports your overall health. Let's turn your home into a haven where you can thrive and live joyfully.

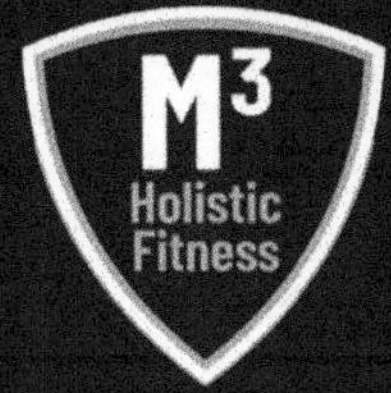

YOUR VIBRANT JOURNEY

Now that you're intimately familiar with the M3 Method's three best friends – Mindset, Movement, and Meals – you've seen their strengths and the magic they create together.

This powerful trio isn't just a formula; it's a lifestyle, a vibrant weaving through the fabric of your life. So, what's next? How do you integrate this newfound wisdom into a life that's not just long but radiantly alive?

Redefining Longevity

Let's redefine longevity. This journey with the M3 Method isn't about turning back the hands of time. It's about ensuring those hands move at a pace that allows you to savor every moment, every milestone. We're aiming for a life where quality meets quantity, where each day is rich with experiences. It's about waking up every morning with energy and enthusiasm, ready to take on the world, and going to bed each night with a sense of fulfillment. This means making conscious choices every day that support your health, from the food you eat to the way you move your body to the thoughts you think.

Growth Mindset

How will your growth mindset influence the years to come? It's a lifelong journey, a consistent effort to build resilience and optimism. Imagine treating mindfulness like a gym membership for your mind, which in return decreases stress, reduces health risks, and leads to a happier life. How will you challenge your views and learn from your experiences starting today?

Begin by setting daily goals that match your aspirations. Make it a habit to appreciate the good in your life, keeping your spirits high. Dive into activities that challenge your intellect, whether tackling a new book, solving puzzles, or picking up a new skill. Keep company with people who lift you up and inspire you and pay attention to the energy you bring to every space you enter. A strong mindset is about crafting a mental space that helps you excel, no matter the challenges ahead.

The Rhythm of Life

Movement in the M3 Method is like a soundtrack to your life, setting the rhythm for your days. What new actions will you embrace? Will it be the liberating spins of a dance class or the serene flow of a yoga session? Remember, movement in the M3 Method is a way to honor your body and spirit. It's a lifestyle choice, one that your future self will look back on with gratitude.

Think of movement as more than exercise. It's about staying active throughout your day. Take the stairs instead of the elevator, walk or bike instead of driving short distances, and find joy in activities that get you moving. Try different forms of exercise to keep things interesting and find what you love. Incorporate strength training, cardio, flexibility, and balance exercises into your routine to keep your body functioning optimally. Movement should be enjoyable, something you

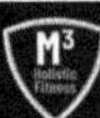

look forward to, and that leaves you feeling energized and refreshed.

The Art of Nourishing

In the M3 Method, thinking about meals goes way beyond just eating right—it's about making everything you do a part of your nourishment. Think of yourself as the head chef in your own life's kitchen. Sure, you pick out great ingredients for your body, but what about food for your soul? The things you love doing, the people who make you smile, and those relaxing moments just for you are all on the menu too.

When you're whipping up meals, go for whole foods packed with nutrients that keep you feeling great. Have fun in the kitchen trying out new recipes and really enjoy the flavors and the process. Make eating a time to connect with family and friends, which strengthens your relationships. And don't forget to do things that feed your spirit. Whether it's picking up a new hobby, spending time outside, or just curling up with a good book, it's all part of living a well-rounded, joyful life. After all, a good life is like a great meal—it's all about enjoying every bite.

Opportunities and Possibilities

The path ahead is filled with chances to dive into the M3 Method. Think of it as your guide to a life that's not just longer, but richer and full of zest. This journey is all about tackling challenges head-on, mixing up your routine, and making connections that make life better.

Why not set some goals that really resonate with what you're passionate about? Try something new that scares you a little—it's all part of the adventure. Gather a crew of folks who get it, and who share your enthusiasm for a healthy, energetic lifestyle. And keep your mind open to learning. Every

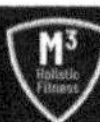

hurdle you come across is a chance to grow stronger and smarter. It's your adventure—make it vibrant and meaningful!

Gear Up for the Best Years

Your best years are just around the corner! With the M3 Method in your toolkit, you're well-equipped to make these years truly count. How do you plan to use what you've learned to shape a life that's not only longer but full of energy, purpose, and joy?

Why not start today? Maybe you'll set a new fitness goal, try out a fresh, healthy recipe, or take a moment to appreciate what you have. Your journey with the M3 Method is deeply personal and packed with potential. Here's to embracing every moment with determination and enthusiasm. Ready to dive in? Scan this QR code or visit our website to begin your vibrant journey.

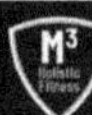

MEALS ACTIONS

Review the following activities and complete at least three of them to help you integrate the Movement content into your life. Bonus points if you accomplish all of them.

1. Mindful Eating Diary: Start a mindful eating diary. For one week, note down your experiences with being present during meals, focusing on the flavors, textures, and how each meal makes you feel.

2. Energizing Nutrient Challenge: For the next 30 days, include at least one energizing nutrient in every meal. Share your favorite energizing meal recipes with friends or on social media.

3. Digestive Health Plan: Create a two-week plan to improve your digestive health. Include probiotics, fiber-rich foods, and ample water in your diet. Document the changes in your digestion and overall well-being.

4. Sustainable Eating Initiative: Commit to making sustainable food choices for a month. This could include eating local and organic foods, reducing food waste, or trying plant-based meals.

5. Cooking at Home Challenge: Cook all your meals at home for a week. Experiment with new recipes that align with the MEALS principles and share your culinary creations online.

6. Hydration Tracker: Track your water intake for 30 days, aiming for the recommended daily amount. Note any changes in energy levels, skin, and overall health.

7. Educational Food Documentary Night: Host a movie night (virtually or in-person) with friends or family to watch a documentary about nutrition and discuss it afterward.

8. Balance & Quality Food Journal: Keep a food journal for two weeks, focusing on balance and quality. Reflect on how balanced and high-quality meals affect your mood and energy levels.

9. Nutrition Webinar or Workshop: Attend a nutrition webinar or workshop to deepen your knowledge about holistic nutrition. Share your learnings and insights with your community.

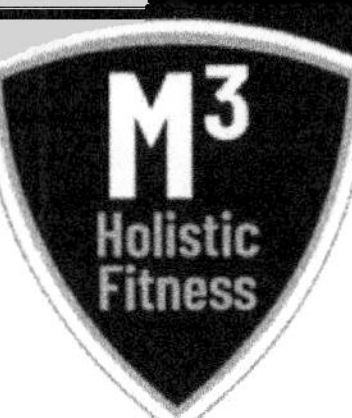

WHAT DOES *YOUR* LIFE LOOK LIKE?

1. Place a dot in each category to indicate your level of satisfaction within each area. A dot at the **center of the circle to indicate dissatisfaction**, or towards the **outer edge to indicate satisfaction**. Most people fall somewhere in between. (see example)

2. Connect the dots to see your **M3 Circle of Life.**

3. Identify imbalances. Determine where to spend more time and energy to create balance. **This will help you create a better balance for your best Badass Life.**

SATISFACTION

DISSATISFACTION

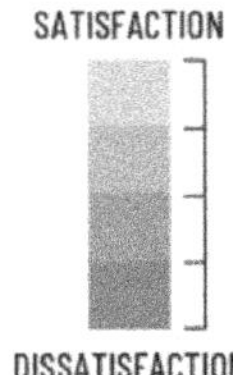

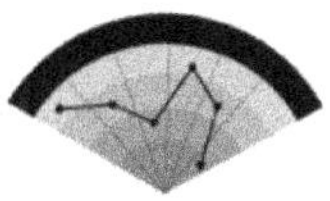

EXAMPLE

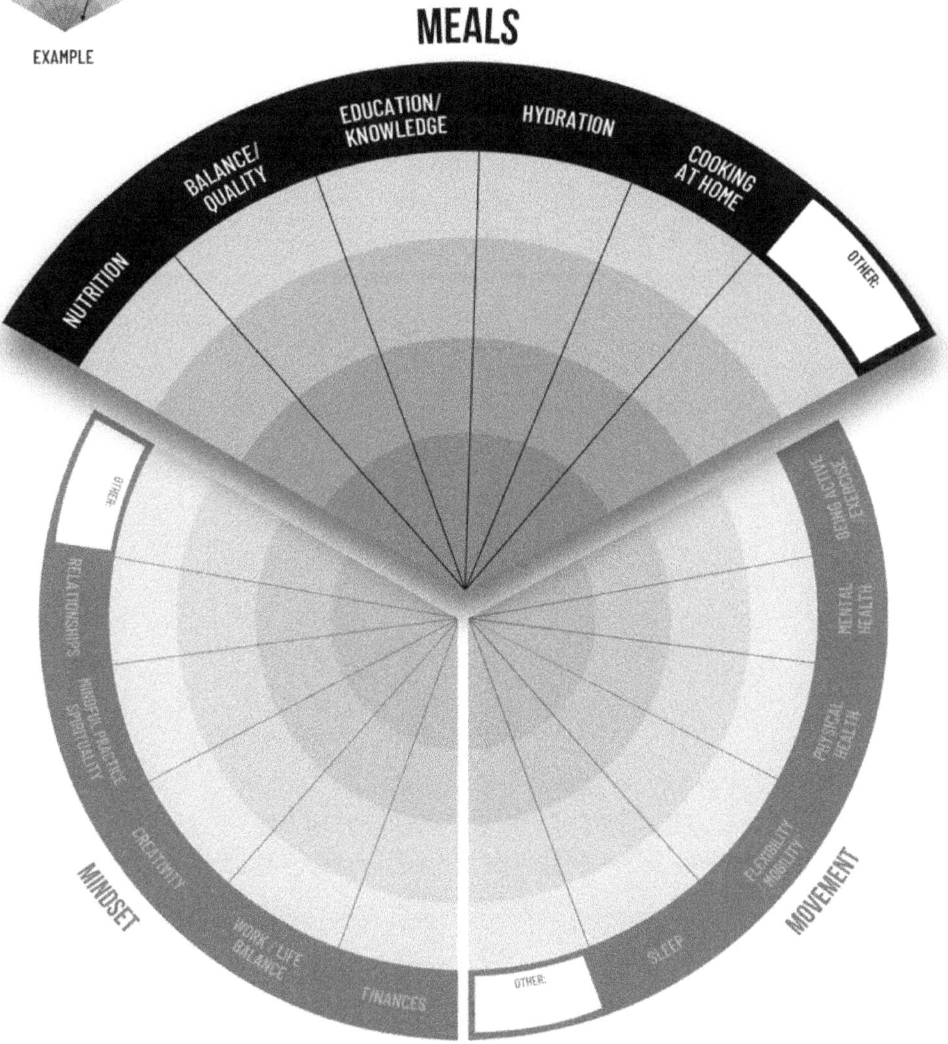

MEALS

FREE DOWNLOAD

M3 Circle of Life Worksheet

http://dirkschultz.com/circle-of-life

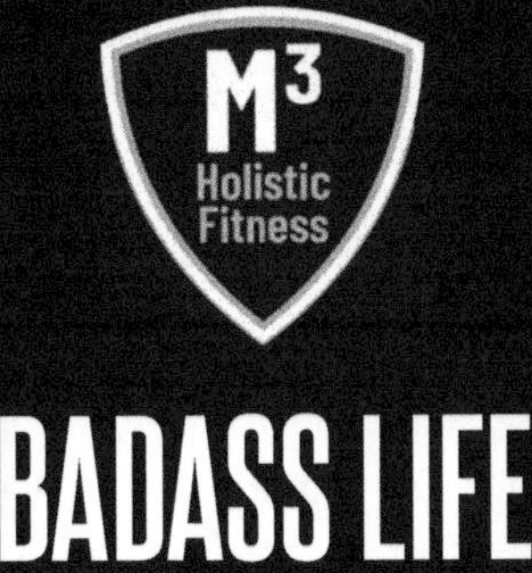

BADASS LIFE

Creating Your BADASS LIFE

*"The only thing standing between you and your goal
is the bullshit story you keep telling yourself
as to why you can't achieve it."
~The Wolf of Wall Street*

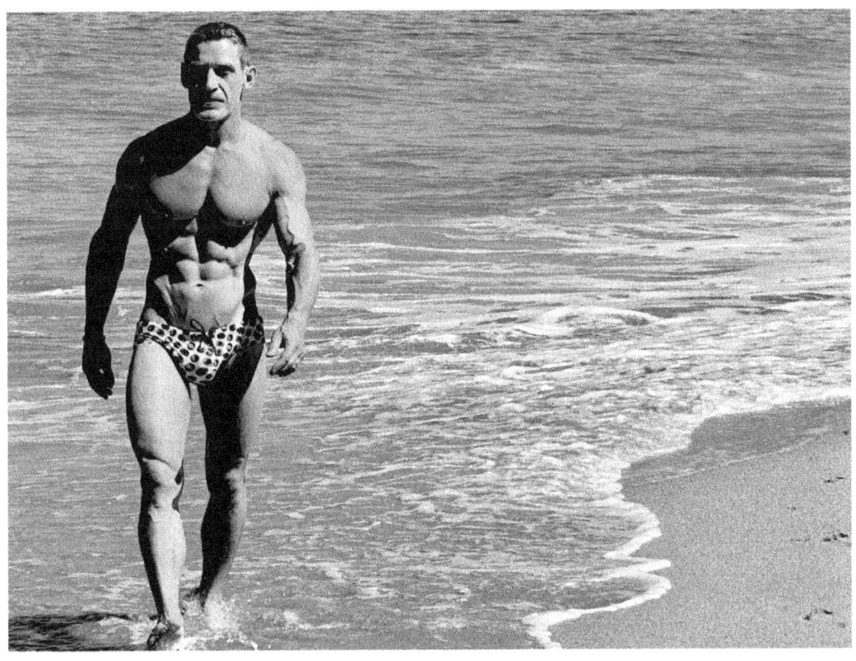

The M3 Method goes beyond simply achieving an integrated, holistic life. It serves as a powerful affirmation when you look in the mirror, recognizing that you're a BADASS gay man committed to making this significant chapter the best years of your life.

Now that we've been on this epic ride together, learning about the M3 Method and how it can transform your life, hold onto your hats, because it's time to level up and turn that life of your new M3 Mindset into a bona fide BADASS LIFE?

You've already got the M3 Method under your belt. That's your toolbox, your Jedi training, your life's cheat codes, whatever you want to call it. Now, let's transform that wisdom into something extraordinary. The BADASS life you're about to create is bursting with enthusiasm, backed by an attitude that empowers, full of determination, fueled by ambition, grounded in self-belief, and fortified with the stamina to go the distance.

Let's break it down, shall we? Mindset is where your Badass Life kicks off. It's the meeting point of a killer attitude and sky-high ambition. It's where you start seeing challenges as opportunities and setbacks as lessons. Your ambition isn't just a wish; it's your roadmap, laying out exactly how you'll conquer every obstacle and seize every chance to grow, whether that's in your workouts, your meals, or even your downtime.

When it comes to Movement, that's where you flex your determination and build stamina. It's one thing to have the intention of leading an active life; it's a whole other game to lace up those sneakers and hit the pavement, day in, day out. But this isn't just about physical stamina. Remember, your mind needs workouts too, to keep you resilient and bouncing back from whatever life throws your way.

Meals are where it gets real. We've been talking about meals 'On the Plate,' but remember our discussions about

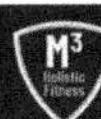

meals 'Off the Plate'? In your BADASS life, meals go beyond what you're eating for lunch. This is holistic nourishment—something that includes not just the food you consume but also the relationships you nurture, the books you devour, and the hobbies that feed your soul. This is about the nourishment that fuels every facet of your being, making you a well-rounded, unstoppable force of nature.

Alright, let's weave that "BADASS" right into our M3 framework because, trust me, they're like two puzzle pieces that snap together perfectly.

B.A.D.A.S.S.

B | Bursting Enthusiasm: Remember when we talked about cultivating a vibrant Mindset? That's where your enthusiasm finds its fuel. You can't go far without passion, and once you direct that toward your goals, you're basically unstoppable.

A | Attitude that Empowers: Your Mindset also shapes your attitude, coloring how you see and interact with the world. That's the power of positive thinking, my friend! And in your BADASS life, it's non-negotiable.

D | Determination to Succeed: These dovetails perfectly with Movement. You need that rock-solid determination to get you through the toughest yoga class, the longest run, or even just a day when the couch looks a little too inviting.

A | Ambition that Fuels Your Dreams: Think of this as your Mindset's long game. Your ambitions are your North Star, guiding everything from your daily actions to your lifelong plans. They're the fire under your... well, you get it.

S | Self-Belief: This one's crucial and ties into our Meals category, especially when we're talking about meals 'Off the Plate.' Your self-belief is what allows you to make nourishing choices for your body and soul without a shred of guilt. It's the underpinning of every smart choice you make, every risk you take, and every goal you smash.

S | Stamina to Go the Distance: We touched on this one under Movement, but it's worth repeating. Stamina isn't just for marathons or endurance sports. It's also the grit and resilience that help you bounce back, adapt, and keep pushing toward what you want.

When M3 and BADASS join forces, you don't just get a life—you get a life that's teeming with enthusiasm, powered by an unshakable attitude, propelled by sheer determination and lofty ambitions, anchored in unyielding self-belief, and armed with the stamina to brave any challenge. This, my friend, is your BADASS LIFE, and it's not merely about longevity. It's about living each moment with a richness and fullness that make the years irrelevant.

Your BADASS LIFE is your masterwork in progress, the sum total of everything you are and aim to be. It's a symphony orchestrated by you, with each section—Mindset, Movement, and Meals—contributing to the crescendo. This isn't a sprint to a finish line but a fascinating, zigzagging journey where the twists and turns are as enriching as the milestones.

How do you go about composing this masterpiece? You start by laying the foundation of unshakeable self-belief, empowering you to make guilt-free, nourishing choices for your body. From there, you weave in the emotional fabric of your life—meaningful relationships that uplift you and extend your vitality. And don't underestimate the power of your attitude toward these life-enriching "Meals." Seeing them as opportunities to refuel both your physical and intellectual self can shift your daily habits toward choices that add not just years to your life but life to your years.

The path ahead also beckons you toward intellectual nourishment, urging you to devour books, engage in thought-provoking dialogues, or take skill-building courses. It's like feed-

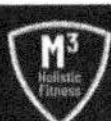

ing protein to your brain! Add a dash of self-development, whether it's through mindfulness practice, diving into hobbies, or engaging in activities that boost your self-esteem, and you're well on your way to a life that is not just well-lived but gloriously BADASS.

So, are you ready to make this chapter the most exhilarating one yet? Your BADASS LIFE is calling, and it's tailored to your unique goals, tastes, and lifestyle. It's all about balance, purposeful choices, and staying true to your core values. Take the M3 Method to heart, let it be your compass, and start carving out your journey to holistic fitness and well-being. Because remember, the journey itself is what makes your life truly BADASS. Strap in; your most incredible adventure is just a heartbeat away.

What are you waiting for? It's time to TAKE ACTION...

A·C·T·I·O·N

A | Align with your vision: Make your vision a daily habit. Own it, visualize it, feel it, and embody it. Visualize your goals and success regularly to stay focused and motivated on your journey.

C | Conquer your fears: Don't let fear hold you back. Face your fears head-on, identify where they come from, and change your relationship with them. As the saying goes, "Face your fears and do it anyway." Remember that fear and excitement originate from the same place, so flip the script and replace fear with excitement.

T | Team up with supportive people: Share your goals with your family, friends, mentors, and those who genuinely support and hold you accountable. These are the folks who uplift you and celebrate your journey and achievements with true enthusiasm.

I | Invest in yourself: Dedicate your time, money, and energy to propel yourself forward and make your vision a reality. Prioritize self-improvement, education, and self-care to lay a solid foundation for your success.

O | Organize your plan: Put your plan down in detail, breaking it into manageable steps. Review it daily to ensure you stay on track and be ready to adapt when necessary.

N | Navigate your next best move and seize the moment: Choose one or two actions to commit to and take them now. Remember that any forward movement, regardless of its size, generates momentum, and each step matters. You can't adjust your course if you're standing still, so embrace the present and get started now! Enjoy the journey, learn from your experiences, and always remember that the time to act is right now. Have fun along the way!

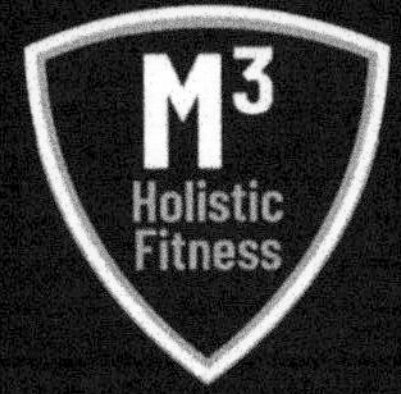

Congratulations! You have completed your tour of the M3 Method and are now ready to begin reinventing your life for the 50+ road ahead.

Now, more than ever, it's important to take a moment to look back on the amazing changes that have taken place. This isn't simply finishing a book; it marks the start of a fresh chapter in your life, where overall well-being and staying fit aren't distant goals but daily experiences. You now have the understanding and resources to incorporate wellness into every part of who you are, crafting a colorful life filled with vitality, joy, and harmony.

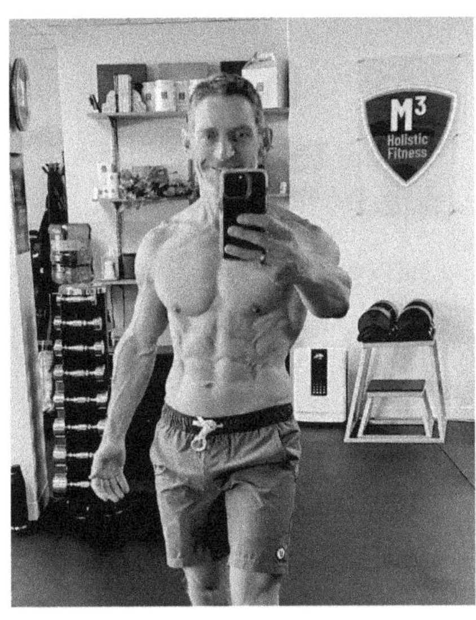

Imagine standing before a mirror, not just looking, but truly seeing the person you've become through this journey. There's a glow of health that radiates from within, a spark in your eyes that speaks of inner peace and contentment. This is the result of more than just physical training; it's the outcome of nurturing relationships that support and uplift you, embracing mindful practices that ground and center you, unleashing creativity that fuels your soul, and finding that delicate balance between work and life that once seemed elusive.

You've learned to navigate your finances with wisdom and foresight, turning what might have been a source of stress into a foundation of security and freedom. You've discovered the transformative power of good sleep hygiene, waking up each day with energy and clarity. And with a clear vision, you've charted a course toward your dreams, armed with the belief in your power to achieve them.

This sense of personal pride and accomplishment isn't just about what you've achieved externally; it's about the internal growth that has taken place. You've sculpted yourself into someone who faces life with resilience, adaptability, and a positive mindset. The challenges and obstacles that life inevitably throws your way are no longer insurmountable; they are opportunities for growth and learning.

As you move forward from here, remember that the principles of the M3 Method are not just for a moment but for a lifetime. The journey to holistic health and fitness is ongoing, a perpetual cycle of growth, challenge, and triumph. There will be days of struggle and days of victory, but each day is a step forward in your journey.

So, take a moment to celebrate yourself and your journey. Be proud of what you've created, not just in your body, but in your mind and spirit. You've embarked on one of life's greatest adventures—the quest for holistic wellness—and

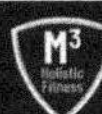

emerged stronger, wiser, and more vibrant. This is not the end; it's a beautiful beginning. The path ahead is yours to shape, with each step guided by the wisdom and strength you've gained. Here's to you, to your health, and to the incredible journey that lies ahead.

NOTES: WHAT DID YOU LEARN FROM THIS CHAPTER?

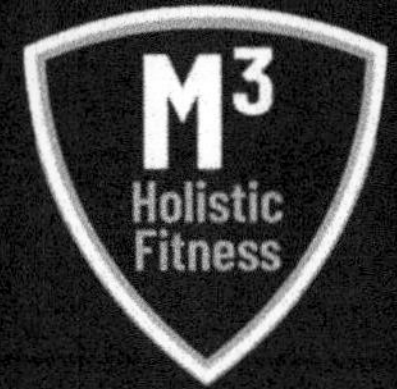

RECAP OF THE M3 METHOD

Let's reflect on everything we've covered about the M3 Method. We've explored Mindset, Movement, and Meals—the three pillars that form the foundation of your BADASS life.

Mindset

We started with mindset because it's the cornerstone of everything. We talked about embracing a growth mindset and how each morning begins with gratitude exercises to keep your positive vibes strong. Setting daily goals isn't just a task—it's a ritual that keeps your ambitions clear. Positive affirmations act as your daily pep talk, reinforcing that unshakeable self-belief. We learned to face fears head-on and to celebrate every win, no matter how small, building resilience and confidence along the way.

Movement

Next, we dove into movement. This isn't just about hitting the gym—it's about integrating movement into your everyday life. You discovered the importance of finding activities you love, whether it's dancing, hiking, or yoga, and making them a regular part of your routine. Mixing up cardio, strength, and flexibility keeps things fresh, and your body engaged. You track your progress, and each journal entry becomes a testament to your commitment. Strength-building exercises, combined with cardio sessions, keep your heart healthy and muscles strong. Stretching and yoga enhance your flexibility, helping you move through life with ease.

Meals

Then, we focused on meals. This isn't just about eating; it's about holistic nourishment. We talked about practicing mindful eating by savoring each bite and the importance of staying hydrated. Your diet is rich in whole foods, lean proteins, healthy fats, and a rainbow of fruits and vegetables. But nourishment doesn't stop with food—it's also about the relationships you build, the hobbies you love, and the continuous learning that keeps your mind sharp and soul fulfilled.

Living a **BADASS** Life

Living a BADASS life is the ultimate goal. You're filled with enthusiasm, empowered by a positive attitude, driven by rock-solid determination, and fueled by ambitious dreams. Your self-belief is unwavering, and you have the stamina to tackle any challenge. The M3 Method ensures every aspect of your life aligns with your goals and values, creating a balanced and fulfilling existence.

Taking **ACTION**

Finally, we talked about taking action. Aligning with your vision and making it a daily habit keeps you focused. Visualizing your goals regularly builds excitement and motivation. Facing your fears head-on and replacing them with excitement is key. Surrounding yourself with supportive people who lift you up and hold you accountable is crucial. Investing in yourself—your time, money, and energy—is worth it. Organizing your plan into manageable steps and reviewing it daily keeps you on track. Navigating your next move by committing to actionable steps and embracing the present moment is essential.

So, there you have it—the M3 Method isn't just a fitness program; it's a way of life. By focusing on Mindset, Movement, and Meals, you're creating a balanced, fulfilling lifestyle that celebrates every moment and every challenge. Embrace this journey with enthusiasm and remember that the best years of your life are still ahead. Let's make them count together.

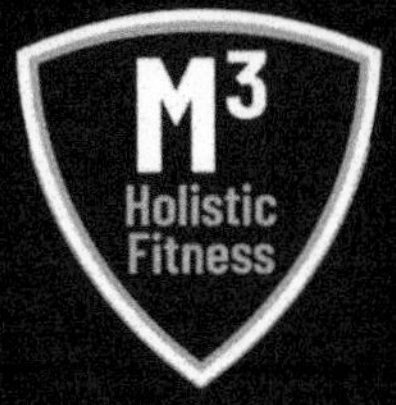

FOUR M3 AGREEMENTS

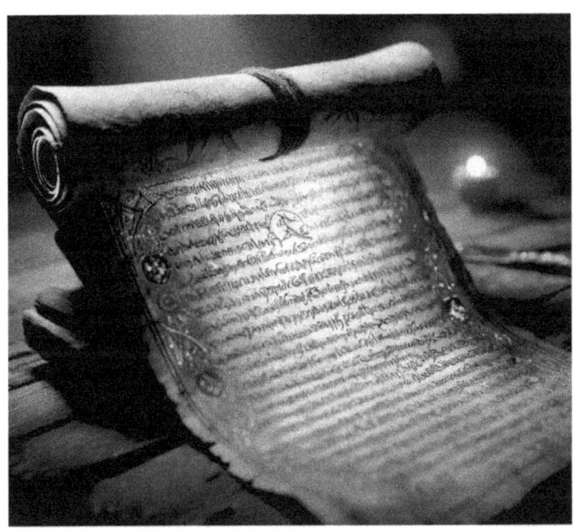

When you join the M3 Holistic Lifestyle, especially as a 50+ gay man with a wealth of experiences, you make four powerful agreements with yourself that will shape your journey toward health, fitness, and overall happiness and well-being. These agreements are tailored to reflect the unique experiences and perspectives of gay men in their prime and revolve around mindset, movement, and meals—the three primary pillars of the M3 Method. Let's explore these agreements in detail.

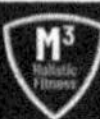

1 — Mindset Agreement

The first agreement you make is to commit to developing a growth mindset. It's about envisioning what you want for your life and embracing a "can do" attitude, free from past societal prejudices or limitations. Remember, you're doing this for yourself, and with the perspective of a 50+ gay man, you have an enriched understanding of self-worth. Find your "why," that burning reason, and make yourself one of your biggest priorities. This agreement isn't just about resilience; it's about celebrating the wisdom and authenticity that comes with your experiences.

2 — Movement Agreement

The second agreement revolves around movement. As a 50+ gay man, the importance of moving with intention, both physically and emotionally, cannot be understated. Recognize that mental health is as vital as physical health. Embrace forms of movement that resonate with your life's journey, whether it's walking, yoga, dancing, swimming, strength training, or any other form of aerobic activity. It's not just about staying active; it's about expressing your authentic self through every movement.

3 — Meals Agreement

The third agreement focuses on meals and is about more than just nutrition. As someone who has lived through diverse experiences, the meals you've enjoyed tell a story—of tradition, celebration, and identity. Commit to nourishing both your body and your spirit and recognize the deep connection between the food you consume and the memories and feelings they evoke.

OFF THE PLATE: Develop and embrace the other areas of your life that will nourish you and feed you off the plate.

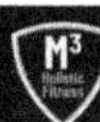

These are areas such as our relationships, careers, spirituality, creativity, and physical activity, to name a few. Finding and feeding these areas is crucial for a holistic well-balanced lifestyle.

4 — Tribe Agreement

The fourth agreement centers on embracing your community and tribe. At this stage in life, especially as a gay man, you understand the importance of unity and shared experiences. This agreement is about actively seeking and nurturing connections with others who resonate with your journey. It's a pledge to both be a source of support and to lean on your chosen family when needed. By intertwining with your community, the M3 Method becomes more than just a personal endeavor; it's a collective movement towards holistic well-being. Remember, together, you thrive.

By making these agreements with yourself, you embark on a holistic journey towards a vibrant and meaningful life as a 50+ gay man. The M3 Method empowers you to develop a growth mindset, move with intention, and nourish yourself both physically and mentally. With each agreement, you align yourself with the path of self—discovery, self—care, and self—actualization.

Keeping your agreements with yourself is of utmost importance on your journey towards holistic well-being. When you commit to develop a growth mindset, move with intention, and nourish yourself both physically and mentally, you are honoring yourself and your journey. By staying true to these agreements, you build self—trust, integrity, and resilience.

Consistency in keeping these agreements reinforces positive habits, propels your progress, and reinforces your belief in your ability to create positive change. When you prioritize yourself and hold yourself accountable to your own promises, you send a powerful message to the world and reaffirm your worthiness of a vibrant and fulfilling life. Remember, you are worthy of the commitment you make to yourself, and by honoring these agreements, you are taking a significant step towards living your best life as a 50+ gay man.

Are you ready to embrace these agreements and embark on a transformational journey that celebrates the prime of your life? Let's dive deeper into the M3 Method and uncover the practical steps and strategies that will guide you toward holistic well-being.

Sign and commit to these agreements:

Signature: _________________________ Date: ______________

Follow Dirk on Instagram: @dirkfitm3

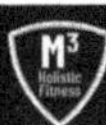

Everlasting Dream

In a world where youth is prized, we've got a secret to be realized. We're gay; we're gray and very fit; at fifty-plus, we're owning it!

We've traded disco for Pilates, but we still know how to shake our bodies. With silver hair and strong biceps, we prove that age is just a song.

From yoga mats to morning jogs, we outpace all those younger dogs. We rock our wrinkles with pride and grace, and there's still plenty of sparkle in this face.

Our diets are clean, and our spirits are high. As we lift those weights and flex with glee, our muscles sing:

"Look at me!"

Parties now start at six, not ten, And we're home in bed by half past then. But don't mistake us for slowing down; we're the fittest 50+ men in town.

With wisdom sharp and laughter free, we've embraced our years with zest and glee. Who needs a fountain of youth to find? We've got our M3 Method to unwind.

So, here's to being fabulous, fit, and gray, to loving life in every way. At fifty and beyond, we reign supreme, Living our gay, gray, and fit everlasting dream!

~David Lloyd Strauss

FINAL MESSAGE FROM DIRK

Hello, my friends,

As we reach the end of this first step in our journey together, I hope you've found inspiration, practical advice, and a renewed sense of purpose.

We've talked about the challenges and triumphs that come with embracing a holistic approach to fitness and well-being, especially as we cross into our 50s and beyond. In a community that often values youth and physical attractiveness, it can be challenging to maintain a sense of self-worth and appeal. But the truth is, the years ahead can be the most rewarding, full of vitality, joy, and purpose.

The ultimate responsibility for your health rests on your shoulders. Coaches and trainers can only do so much; your true mental and physical transformation requires personal investment. And here's the silver lining—it's an engaging, even enjoyable journey when you have the proper structure and accountability in place.

This brings us to the M3 Method. Designed as a holistic lifestyle approach, proper fitness isn't just a physical endeavor. It's a self-reflective journey that starts with a tailored plan covering not just the physical but also the emotional, mental, and spiritual aspects of life. This isn't just about brawn but a full-spectrum life transformation.

At the core of the M3 Method are three pillars: Mindset, Movement, and Meals. The path to well-being isn't just through your muscles; it's a journey within. The M3 Method aims to clear away the obstacles that hinder you from achieving your fullest potential in every aspect of your life.

Whether you're just starting your fitness journey or already a seasoned athlete, the M3 Method is here to support you in living life on your own terms. Remember, to enhance your life, it's essential to make deliberate adjustments with a clear plan and goals in mind. Trust the M3 Method to help you reach your goals.

As we stand here at the threshold of tomorrow, remember that the best years are still ahead. With the M3 Method as your ally, you're equipped to make these years count. How will you use these tools to shape a life that's not just longer but one that's overflowing with energy, purpose, and joy?

Start today. Take that first step by joining the M3 Community and taking Dirk's M3 Holistic Fitness Challenge. Commit to the M3 lifestyle for health and longevity. Whether it's setting a new fitness goal, trying a new healthy recipe, or simply reflecting on what you're grateful for, this challenge is your gateway to a life overflowing with energy, purpose, and joy.

Your journey with the M3 Method is a personal one, full of potential and transformation. Embrace every moment with heart, courage, and the unwavering spirit of the M3 Method. Let's make these years count together. Join us now and become a part of a vibrant, supportive community dedicated to holistic wellness and vibrant living.

With all my support and encouragement,

Dirk Schultz

Join the Community: DirkSchultz.com

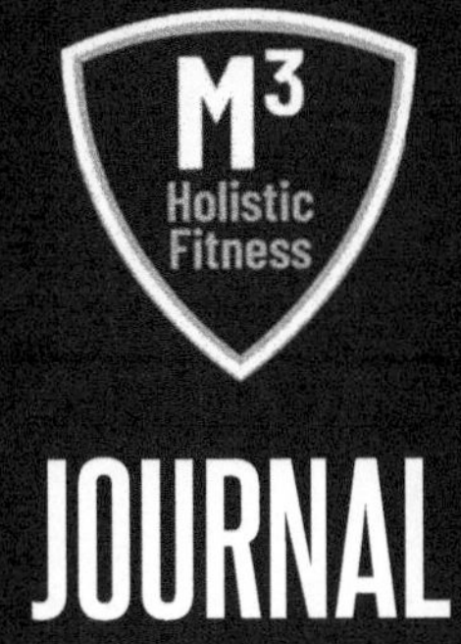

JOURNAL

Order Online | DirkSchultz.com

The M3 Journal is the ultimate playbook where you sketch, plan, and celebrate your journey to becoming the most BADASS version of yourself!

It isn't just a notebook; it's the canvas where you paint the portrait of your most BADASS self. This journal fuses everything we've talked about—the M3 Method and the BADASS lifestyle—into a daily practice that you can literally hold in your hands. Picture it as your life's roadmap, brimming with the colors of Mindset, Movement, and Meals.

Mindset gets its rightful spotlight in this journal. You'll find sections dedicated to your goals, affirmations, and reflections. This is your safe space to jot down the thoughts that uplift you and confront those that hold you back. It's where your mental game gets fine-tuned, helping you embody that bursting enthusiasm and empowering attitude we talked about.

Movement isn't just penciled in—it's highlighted, circled, and underlined. Your M3 Journal comes with pages that encourage you to log your physical activities, whether it's hitting the gym, doing yoga, or going for a nature hike. Here, you channel your determination to succeed and build up the stamina to go the distance. Each entry becomes a badge of honor, showcasing your unwavering commitment to staying active and fierce.

Then there's Meals, and we're talking about nourishment in its broadest sense. In this part of the journal, you capture everything that fuels you. From the food you eat to the relationships you nurture; you'll have designated space to reflect on the elements that enrich your life. This is where you dig deep into the self-belief that grounds you and the ambition that fuels your dreams.

Beyond the triple M's, your M3 Journal will have prompts that foster continuous self-development. It's the nudge you need to engage in intellectual nourishment and emotional growth, tying back into the BADASS qualities you aim to embody.

So, if you're ready to take your life from good to epic, the M3 Journal is your partner in crime. With it, you're not just jotting down words; you're scripting the compelling narrative of your BADASS journey. Consider this journal your daily dose of M3 goodness, an intimate dialogue with yourself that guides, celebrates, and propels you into a life that's as enriching as it is exhilarating.

Grab that pen, my friend. Your BADASS 50+ LIFE is waiting to be written.

Order Now: DirkSchultz.com

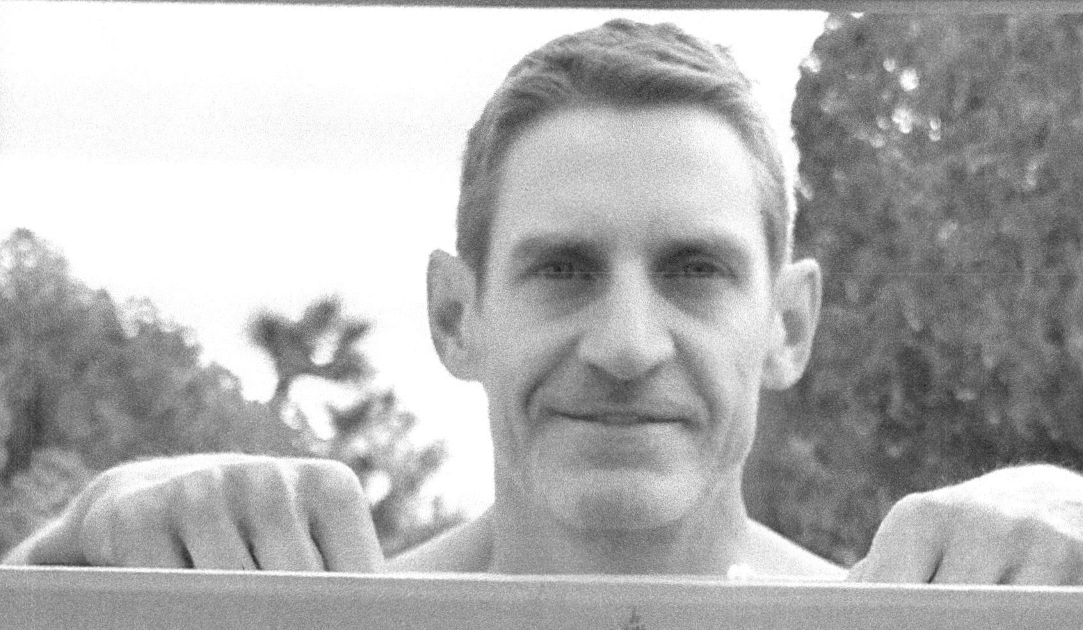
Thank you!

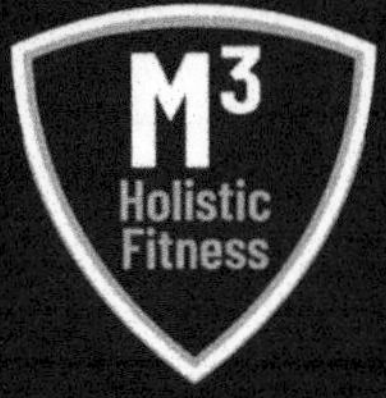

ACKNOWLEDGMENTS

I want to thank the following people who helped this book become a reality.

David Strauss: Friend, writing coach, and mentor

When the idea of writing this book was first presented to me, I thought, 'What do I have to write about?' My ideas and methods of doing things did o't see anything special. Then, as the thought sank in, I thought, 'Why not?' I do have a method of how I train and coach my clients. As I started to flesh out the idea and work with David Strauss, I began to see and feel that my work is valuable and can help people live a holistic, authentic, badass life. I got excited about the process. Working with David led to a few results: I gained more confidence in my work and myself. I started to envision the bigger picture of a book, and perhaps a journal, to accompany it and further people's growth and deepen their learning. I began to think and carry myself differently.

Writing this book helped me create a vision to ramp up my career when I was considering winding down. It gave new life to how I want to spend and serve others in my badass life after 50. Working with David also gave me a broader perspective on what I want to create, including other books I would like to write.

Dave Lusk: My husband

Thank you for all his love and support over the years and during the process of writing this book. Dave has held the space for me as my business shifted from a personal training studio to the expanded M3 Holistic Fitness Studio, sparking the inspiration for the M3 Method and coaching platform, which led to writing this book.

Tony Calucci: Priceless friend

Tony, together with David Strauss, recognized the potential in my work and me. He provided motivation and inspiration and helped generate ideas as I wrote this book. His belief in me was a driving force, continuously propelling me forward in business and in our friendship.

Dawn Shepard: Friend and mentor

I cannot say enough about how grateful I am to Dawn. She said "yes" and hired me at the Aspen Club and Spa when I was an inexperienced trainer. She mentored me then and continues to mentor me today to keep learning about myself and to educate myself in the field of health and wellness. I am so grateful for the opportunities she has provided me and encouraged me to take. Without her, this book would not have been possible.

Lisa Cherney: Mentor and coach.

I have worked with Lisa for years as a mentor and coach. In our time together, Lisa has helped me define what I want my life and business to look like. To create a vision that is bigger

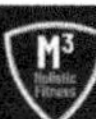

than I could have imagined on my own. To help me identify my limitations and create an action plan to bust through the limiting beliefs and perceived obstacles.

My clients

I have been blessed with amazing BADASS clients who have helped me learn about myself and hone my skills as a health coach and personal trainer. They have taught me as much as I have taught them. I feel blessed every day that I am able to work and create a living with such amazing people.

Parents

My mother and father, who taught me a solid work ethic. To work hard, treat people well, and always be open to continuous self-improvement.

Friends & Family

Thank you to my friends, family, clients, and mentors, and everyone who has helped me in various ways through love, support, lessons, and believing in me.

The Creative Team at We Make Stuff Happen

Wemakestuffhappen.com

Jonathan Christian and Andy Hemsley.

They took my ideas and vision and brought them to life, creating the graphics for this book.

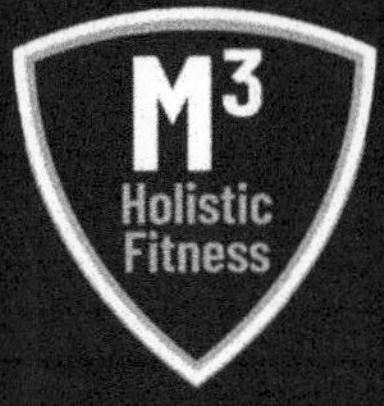

SPECIAL THANKS!

Book Pre-Order Support

Love and gratitude to the following people who pre-ordered this book. Your early support and belief in this project have been a tremendous source of motivation and encouragement.

Your enthusiasm and faith in the value of this work have played a crucial role in bringing this book to life. Each pre-order has not only provided financial backing but also a significant morale boost, reminding me that there is an audience eager to engage with the ideas and stories within these pages.

Thank you for being the first to embark on this journey with me. Your contribution is deeply appreciated and will always be remembered as a foundational part of this book's success.

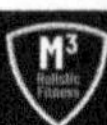

In alphabetical order...

Amy Knight	Kenny Jervis
Ashley Donde	Kevin Pfeiffer
Carla Calucci	Mark Kraft
Chris Perry	Marty Kovacevich
Craig Hartzman	Matt Wogen
Cynthia M Barker	Mike Marron
Dan Katzir	Mitchell Goodman
David Hegarty	Nevada Presley
David Lusk	Paul Feeney
David Stutz	Richelle Pakosz
Dawn Shepard	Rick Dinihanian
Doug Silveira	Robert Reinhart
Erin Lentz	Scooby1961
Frank Hundley	Solomon Robbins
James Campbell	Stephen Bay
Jason Burns	Stephen Szoradi
Jason Morris	Steven Margolin
Jeff Leinbach	Todd Monaghan
Joel Readence	Tony Calucci
Joyce Dara	Tony Cappoli
Kate Lokken	Wendy Feinstein
Kelly Nicholson	William Adams

Endless love and gratitude to each of you!

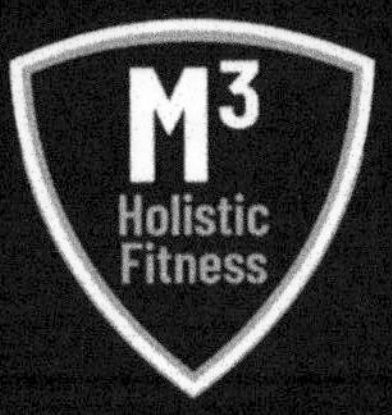

AN ENDORSEMENT FROM TONY C.

I'm Tony Calucci, and I'm thrilled to share my journey with Dirk Schultz and the incredible M3 Method. As a proud member of the M3 Holistic Community for 50+ gay men, I can confidently say that Dirk's approach to fitness and wellness has been nothing short of life changing.

As a 61-year-old man, I have spent many years working out alone, with friends, or with personal trainers. Most of my experiences have been satisfactory. Walk into the gym, exchange pleasantries with friends, and then down to business—the same workouts I have repeated for years with an occasional new exercise thrown in that I saw someone do to try and spice it up! Recently, a friend told me about this trainer here in town, Dirk Schultz, and his incredible M3 Method: Mindset, Movement, and Meals.

When I first started working with Dirk, I was looking for more than just a fitness coach—I was searching for someone who understood the unique challenges and triumphs we face as gay men over 50. From day one, Dirk's vibrant energy, unwavering support, and deep understanding of holistic wellness drew me in. It wasn't long before I realized I had found not just a coach but a friend and mentor.

Dirk spent time getting to know me, my previous workout experiences, my history, injuries, my goals, and my attitude towards my goals and fitness in general. Nothing felt rushed; he wasn't looking at the clock. He was taking notes, looking at me, and asking questions... he was listening!

Once the workouts began, I found his unique approach towards me as an individual to be refreshing and completely focused on my goals, needs, and the best way I could achieve them. I enjoyed the workouts, as hard as they were. I felt good, and I was making progress. He reveled in my success while helping me to understand that my health mindset is the key to my success, making me feel empowered and motivated every step of the way. He introduced me to his M3 Method: Mindset, Movement, and Meals.

What I realized was that he was shifting my mindset during the workout. He was structuring my mindset towards accomplishing the task at hand while keeping me focused on my long-range goals. His amazing understanding of the growth mindset and how it plays an integral part in shaping and assisting you in achieving your goals was extraordinary. This is what puts Dirk in a league of his own with his M3 Method!

As a trainer and life coach, Dirk embodies confidence in his knowledge. He carries an incredibly positive attitude is focused on you as the client with constant feedback while never taking his eyes off your execution of the material he has presented to you. Whether he is tweaking your form or shaping your mind towards accomplishing the task at hand, he is upbeat, engaging, mindful, and intuitive.

Working with Dirk, I've not only seen a transformation in my physical health but also in my mental and emotional well-being. His dedication to helping his clients achieve their best selves is truly inspiring, all while maintaining a fun and supportive atmosphere. His wonderful sense of humor keeps the workouts light and fun... and believe me, we do a lot of laughing!

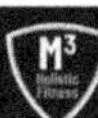

His individualized approach to your physical goals is strongly tied to his passionate understanding of the growth mindset and how it can shape and assist you in achieving your personal goals in and outside of the gym. Your workouts are tailored to you, never boring and never the same! He creates a desire for you to learn and improve. He encourages and draws inspiration from your success. Each workout is specific, fun, challenging yet mindful of your physical limitations while maximizing your effort.

Like no other trainer or coach, he has taught me that the power of one's mindset is a crucial aspect of reaching one's goals in the gym... but more importantly, out of the gym! Our thoughts and beliefs impact our actions and ultimately determine our success or failure. His coaching has impacted my life in and out of the gym!

I had the amazing opportunity to support Dirk behind the scenes, aiding in the creation and review of this book while bouncing around ideas. It was truly an exciting experience! Dirk dedicated his heart and soul to crafting his ideas, offering insights and stories from his experiences.

As time has passed, I have seen transformational changes in myself physically and, more importantly, in my mental approach towards myself and my goals. My friends tell me my physical appearance has been transformed, and it has. The most important journey has been the understanding of the power of an individual's mindset. Dirk has been the impetus for this for me. He stood at the threshold and coached me to a place of success and confidence like no other trainer has done before. This makes him a unique and extraordinary trainer and an inspiring coach!

I really hope this book inspires you to lead a happier, more fulfilling life. The M3 Community is a fantastic group of people who encourage and support each other, and we can't wait for you to be part of it. If you're eager to live a life filled with energy, joy, and resilience, Dirk Schultz and the M3 Method are here to help you make it happen. I assure you; you won't encounter a more committed coach or a more caring community.

Let's make these years our greatest ones—let's do it together! Here's to a vibrant, fit, and fabulous future!

Warm regards,

Tony Calucci

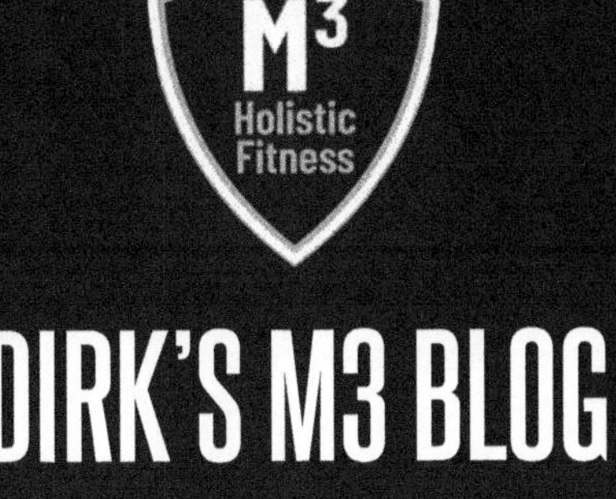

DIRK'S M3 BLOG

Dirk's BLOG: DirkSchultz.com/Blog

Swing by Dirk's blog over at DirkSchultz.com for a good read that'll keep you hooked and moving forward on your wellness journey. It's not just any blog—it's like having a heart-to-heart with an old friend who gets it, especially for us in the 50+ gay crowd looking to live our best lives. From deep dives into the M3 Method that Dirk himself crafted to personal stories and nuggets of wisdom, this blog is where you'll find your dose of inspiration, laughter, and maybe even a kick in the pants when you need it.

So, if you're eager to feel more energized, confident, and connected, Dirk's got you covered. Check it out and see for yourself how each post brings you closer to the vibrant, badass life you're aiming for. I can't wait to see you there!

Flip the next few pages to read
a few of Dirk's recent blog entries.

BLOG
Defying the Myths of Aging

A Journey to Your Best Self

Growing older is a natural part of life, and it comes with its own set of challenges and joys, especially in the gay community where youth and beauty often take center stage. But imagine this: what if your 50s and beyond turn out to be some of the most exhilarating and rewarding years of your life? What if, instead of slowing down, you're just revving up for an incredible new chapter? This is the heart of the M3 Method.

Embracing a New Chapter

Dirk doesn't just talk the talk; he's walked the walk. Entering his 50s as a proud, fit gay man, Dirk has battled through his own journey of self-discovery, overcoming adversity and emerging stronger and more determined. His M3 Method—focused on Mindset, Movement, and Meals—is more than a fitness plan; it's a holistic approach to living that celebrates the wisdom, experience, and maturity that come with age.

The Power of Mindset

One of the most damaging myths about aging is that our best years are behind us. Dirk challenges this head-on, encouraging his clients to adopt a growth mindset that sees potential for joy, achievement, and fulfillment at any age. "Unlocking the best year of your life," as Dirk puts it, begins in the mind. With his guidance, you'll learn to cultivate mindfulness, develop a growth mindset, and connect with your authentic

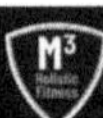

self, all of which are fundamental to living a life that's not only longer but richer and more rewarding.

Movement as a Celebration

Forget the notion that aging means slowing down. The M3 Method encourages movement in all its forms, from high-intensity workouts to peaceful yoga sessions, all tailored to suit your unique needs and preferences. Dirk's approach is about finding joy in activity—celebrating what your body can do rather than lamenting what it can't. He'll help you improve your strength, stability, and mobility, proving that age is no barrier to physical fitness.

Nourishment for Body and Soul

Meals in the M3 Method are about more than just food. They represent a way to nourish your body and soul, with a focus on quality, balance, and the joy of eating. Dirk emphasizes the importance of "feeding yourself better on the plate and off the plate," advocating for a diet that fuels your body while also encouraging you to indulge in the activities and relationships that feed your spirit. This holistic approach to nutrition is about vitality, energy, and enjoying the richness of life.

Building a Supportive Community

One of the most valuable aspects of working with Dirk is the sense of community he fosters. In the journey to defy aging myths, having a tribe that supports and uplifts you is invaluable. Dirk's commitment to creating connections among his clients not only enhances the journey but also reinforces the idea that we're all in this together, exploring what it means to live authentically, out, and proud.

Your Adventure Awaits

Working with Dirk Schultz isn't just about defying aging; it's about redefining it. It's about proving that the 50+ years can be a time of unparalleled growth, joy, and adventure. Through the M3 Method, Dirk offers not just a fitness plan but a blueprint for a life well-lived, inviting you to join him in celebrating every moment, every challenge, and every triumph.

Your adventure is waiting. Are you ready to embark on this journey to your best self with Dirk Schultz? Let's defy the myths of aging together and show the world what it truly means to be gay, gray, and fit after 50.

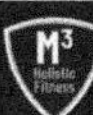

Thriving with the M3 Method

Imagine waking up each day with a surge of energy that carries you through your morning routine, feeling a vitality that radiates from within, and possessing a confidence that illuminates every room you enter. This isn't just a dream; it's the reality for those who have embraced the M3 Method of holistic fitness and wellness, crafted by holistic wellness coach Dirk Schultz. The M3 Method isn't just about adding years to your life; it's about adding life to your years, especially for the 50+ gay community who are redefining what it means to age with grace, power, and sex appeal.

A New Dawn of Energy and Vitality

For many, the concept of aging comes with fears of dwindling energy and fading vitality. However, those who have journeyed with the M3 Method tell a different story. They speak of mornings filled with enthusiasm, days powered by unwavering stamina, and evenings that glow with the satisfaction of a day well-lived. This energy isn't just physical; it's a profound sense of aliveness that permeates every aspect of their being.

Rediscovering Your Sex Appeal

In a culture that often idolizes youth, finding and embracing your sex appeal at 50+ can seem like a daunting task. Yet, Dirk's M3 Method shines a spotlight on the undeniable allure that comes with maturity. It's a sex appeal rooted in self-assurance, the elegance of experience, and the magnetic pull of someone who knows exactly who they are. This isn't about recapturing the past; it's about celebrating the present and looking forward to the future with a confident, sexy stride.

The Unshakable Confidence of Authentic Living

One of the most enriching outcomes of living the M3 Method is the profound confidence it instills. This confidence comes from a deep alignment between your actions and your values, from the pride of taking control of your health and wellness, and from the courage to live authentically. It's a confidence that says, "I am proud of who I am, and I am excited about where I'm going." It's not just felt internally; it's seen by everyone around you.

The Holistic Harmony of Mind, Body, and Spirit

At its core, the M3 Method celebrates the harmonious integration of mind, body, and spirit. It's a holistic approach that recognizes the interconnectivity of our mental, physical, and emotional health. This harmony manifests in a life where stress is managed with grace, where the body is honored and cared for, and where the spirit is nourished by connections, creativity, and purpose.

Beyond the Mirror: The Reflection of a Life Well-Lived

For those who follow the M3 Method, the reflection they see in the mirror is one of vibrant health, radiant energy, and indomitable spirit. But the beauty of this reflection lies not just in what is seen but in what is felt. It's the inner glow of someone who has embraced their journey, who has faced challenges with resilience, and who stands proud in their authenticity.

Life on the other side of living the M3 Method is a testament to the power of holistic wellness. It's a life where ener-

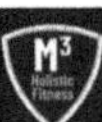

gy, vitality, sex appeal, and confidence are not just aspirations but everyday realities. It's a life where aging is not feared but celebrated as an opportunity for continued growth, exploration, and fulfillment.

Join Dirk Schultz and discover the transformative power of the M3 Method. Let's reimagine what it means to live well, proving that the best is yet to come.

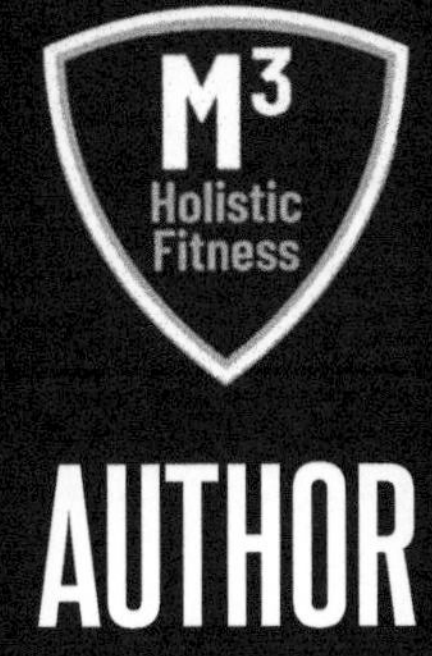

AUTHOR

About Dirk Schultz

Dirk Schultz, stepping confidently into his 50s as a proud gay man, carries with him a life story marked by resilience and profound transformation. His early experiences, shadowed by abuse and abandonment, led him to find refuge and strength in fitness. This journey, initially a symbol of external resilience, evolved into an avenue for deep inner empowerment, helping Dirk to break free from the burdens of his past.

For Dirk, and many like him in the gay community, the challenge of aging brings unique complexities, especially in a culture that often idolizes youth and physical attractiveness. As Dirk's own journey unfolded, his values and relationships deepened, mirroring the journey of many gay men in their 50s who seek to rediscover their self-worth and reignite their social and sexual appeal.

Dirk is a firm believer in taking charge of your health and well-being. He knows that personal dedication plays a key role in the path to wellness. This belief inspired him to develop the M3 Method, a well-rounded approach to fitness and life. His method isn't just about exercise; it embraces emotional, mental, and spiritual wellness, aiming for a complete personal transformation.

The M3 Method, built on the foundation of Mindset, Movement, and Meals, reflects Dirk's unique take on fitness. It's a journey of self-discovery that he has honed over his many years in the fitness world starting back in 2004. Drawing from his diverse experience in reputable fitness clubs and certifications from well-known institutions, Dirk offers a treasure trove of wisdom and a tailored touch to his wellness programs.

Dirk Schultz's mission is to empower individuals, whether they are fitness beginners or seasoned athletes, to take control of their lives with intention and purpose. He emphasizes the importance of strategic, intentional changes backed by measurable outcomes. Through the M3 Method, Dirk Schultz offers more than a fitness program; he offers a pathway to a transformative way of life, guiding others to find their strength and live authentically at any age.